SOCIETE INTERNATIONALE D'UROLOGIE REPORTS

Oncogenes and Molecular Genetics of Urological Tumours

SOCIETE INTERNATIONALE D'UROLOGIE REPORTS

Oncogenes and Molecular Genetics of Urological Tumours

Edited by

C. A. Olsson
Professor, Department of Urology, Columbia University
College of Physicians and Surgeons, New York, USA

CHURCHILL LIVINGSTONE
EDINBURGH LONDON MADRID MELBOURNE NEW YORK AND TOKYO 1992

CHURCHILL LIVINGSTONE
Medical Division of Longman Group UK Limited

Distributed in the United States of America by
Churchill Livingstone Inc., 650 Avenue of the Americas, New York, N.Y. 10011, and by associated companies, branches and representatives throughout the world.

First published 1992

ISBN 0-443-04646-8

British Library Cataloguing in Publication Data
A catalogue record for this book is available from the British Library.

Library of Congress Cataloging in Publication Data is available.

Typeset by BP Integraphics Ltd., Bath, Avon
Printed in Great Britain at The Bath Press Ltd., Bath, Avon

Contents

Contributors

R. Ackermann
Department of Urology, University of Düsseldorf Medical School, Düsseldorf, Germany

G. L. Adessi
Unite de Biochimie Hormonale et des régulations, Besançon, France

N. J. Agnantis
Hellenic Anticancer Institute, Athens, Greece

L. Andersson
Department of Urology, Karolinska Hospital, Stockholm, Sweden

Y. Asano
Department of Urology, Hokkaido University School of Medicine, Sapporo, Japan

U. S. R. Bergerheim
Department of Urology, Karolinska Hospital, Stockholm, Sweden

H. Bittard
Service d'Urologie, Besançon, France

M. Bittard
Service d'Urologie, Besançon, France

A. V. Bono
Department of Urology and Cytogenetics, University Hospital, Varese, Italy

M. J. G. Bussemakers
Department of Urology, University Hospital Nijmegen, Nijmegen, The Netherlands

R. Buttyan
Department of Urology, Columbia University, College of Physicians and Surgeons, New York, USA

J. C. Carrasco-Aznar
Urology Unit, Córdoba University Medical School and Reina Sofia University Hospital, Córdoba, Spain

R. Casalone
Department of Urology and Cytogenetics, University Hospital, Varese, Italy

G. E. Chechile
IUNA Fundacion Puigvert, Barcelona, Spain

G. D. Chisholm
University Department of Surgery/Urology, Western General Hospital, Edinburgh, Scotland

D. S. Coffey
The Johns Hopkins University School of Medicine, Baltimore, Maryland, USA

V. P. Collins
Ludwig Institute for Cancer Research; Karolinska Hospital; Gothenbergs University, Stockholm, Sweden

R. Connelly
The Cleveland Clinic Foundation, Cleveland, USA

M. Colombel
Department of Urology, Columbia University, College of Physicians and Surgeons, New York, USA

A. Cranidis
Department of Urology, Medical School, University of Crete, Heraklion, Crete, Greece

F. M. J. Debruyne
Department of Urology, University Hospital Nijmegen, Nijmegen, The Netherlands

D. Delakas
Medical School, University of Crete, Heraklion, Crete, Greece

F. Descotes
Unité de Biochimie Hormonale et des régulations, Besançon, France

C. Dimopoulos
Departments of Urology and Pathology, Athens University Medical School, Athens, Greece

P. J. Effert
Division of Urology, Duke University School of Medicine, North Carolina; Department of Medicine and the Curriculum in Genetics, Lineberger Comprehensive Cancer Center, UNC School of Medicine, North Carolina, USA

Y. Endo
Department of Experimental Therapeutics, Cancer Research Institute, Kanazawa University, Kanazawa, Japan

D. Filaktopoulos
Departments of Urology and Pathology, Athens University Medical School, Athens, Greece

R. A. Frye
Department of Medicine and the Curriculum in Genetics, Lineberger Comprehensive Cancer Center, UNC School of Medicine, North Carolina, USA

K. Fujimoto
National Cancer Center, Chuo-ku, Tokyo, Japan

Y. Furuya
Department of Urology, School of Medicine, Chiba University, Chiba, Japan

Z. L. Ge
Institute of Urology, Beijing Medical University, Beijing, China

P. Granata
Department of Urology and Cytogenetics, University Hospital, Varese, Italy

F. L. Gu
Institute of Urology, Beijing Medical University, Beijing, China

M. Hamada
Department of Urology, Hokkaido University School of Medicine, Sapporo, Japan

T. Hasegawa
Department of Urology, School of Medicine, Kanazawa University, Kanazawa, Japan

H. Hisazumi
Department of Urology, School of Medicine, Kanazawa University, Kanazawa, Japan

A. Ichihara
Institute for Enzyme Research, Tokushima University, Tokushima, Japan

T. Inai
Department of Urology, School of Medicine, Tokushima University, Tokushima, Japan

W. B. Isaacs
The Johns Hopkins University School of Medicine, Baltimore, Maryland, USA

S. Kagawa
Department of Urology, School of Medicine, Tokushima University, Tokushima, Japan

Y. Kakehi
Department of Urology, Faculty of Medicine, Kyoto University, Kyoto, Japan

T. Kakizoe
National Cancer Center Hospital, Chuo-ku, Tokyo, Japan

H. Kanayama
Department of Urology, School of Medicine, Tokushima University, Tokushima, Japan

K. Kazuto
Department of Urology, School of Medicine, Kanazawa University, Kanazawa, Japan

E. Khenifar
Service d'Urologie, Besançon, France

A. Khihara
Institute for Enzyme Research, Tokushima University, Tokushima, Japan

E. A. Klein
The Cleveland Clinic Foundation, Cleveland, USA

T. Koyanagi
Department of Urology, Hokkaido University School of Medicine, Sapporo, Japan

K. Kurokawa
Department of Urology, School of Medicine, Tokushima University, Tokushima, Japan

H. Levin
The Cleveland Clinic Foundation, Cleveland, USA

E. T. Liu
Department of Medicine and the Curriculum in Genetics, Lineberger Comprehensive Cancer Center, UNC School of Medicine, North Carolina, USA

A. Lopez-Beltran
Pathology Unit, Córdoba University Medical School and Reina Sofia University Hospital, Córdoba, Spain

R. Lopez-Pardo
Urology Unit, Córdoba University Medical School and Reina Sofia University Hospital, Córdoba, Spain

A. Maru
Jinyukai Urological Hospital, Sumikawa, Sapporo, Japan

C. Morales-Jimenez
Pathology Unit, Córdoba University Medical School and Reina Sofia University Hospital, Córdoba, Spain

T. Mori
Department of Urology, Hokkaido University School of Medicine, Sapporo, Japan

S. Nakanishi
Jinyukai Urological Hospital, Sumikawa, Sapporo, Japan

L. Nakopoulou
Departments of Urology and Pathology, Athens University Medical School, Athens, Greece

A. Neubauer
Department of Medicine and the Curriculum in Genetics, Lineberger Comprehensive Cancer Center, UNC School of Medicine, North Carolina, USA

M. Noguchi
Department of Experimental Therapeutics, Cancer Research Institute, Kanazawa University, Kanazawa, Japan

O. Ogawa
Department of Urology, Faculty of Medicine, Kyoto University, Kyoto, Japan

C. A. Olsson
Professor, Department of Urology, Columbia University College of Physicians and Surgeons, New York, USA

J. Parliaras
Institute of Biological Research and Biotechnology, National Hellenic Research Foundation, Athens, Greece

A. Remy-Martin
Unité de Biochimie Hormonale et des régulations, Besançon, France

C. Reymundo
Pathology Unit, Córdoba University Medical School and Reina Sofia University Hospital, Córdoba, Spain

B. Saitoh
Jinyukai Urological Hospital, Sumikawa, Sapporo, Japan

M. Santamaria Ossorio
Biochemistry Unit, Córdoba University Medical School and Reina Sofia University Hospital, Córdoba, Spain

T. Sasaki
Department of Experimental Therapeutics, Cancer Research Institute, Kanazawa University, Kanazawa, Japan

N. Sato
Department of Urology, School of Medicine, Chiba University, Chiba, Japan

J. A. Schalken
Urological Research Laboratory, University Hospital Nijmegen, Nijmegen, The Netherlands

M. Schumer
Division of Urology, Maimonides Medical Center, Brooklyn, New York, USA

J. C. Shen
Institute of Urology, Beijing Medical University, Beijing, China

J. Shimazaki
Department of Urology, School of Medicine, Chiba University, Chiba, Japan

N. Shinohara
Department of Urology, Hokkaido University School of Medicine, Sapporo, Japan

D. A. Spandidos
Medical School, University of Crete and Institute of Biological Research and Biotechnology, National Hellenic Research Foundation, Athens, Greece

T. Strohmeyer
Department of Urology, University of Düsseldorf Medical School, Düsseldorf, Germany

T. Takamatsu
Jinyukai Urological Hospital, Sumikawa, Sapporo, Japan

I. Takeuchi
Department of Urology, Hokkaido University School of Medicine, Sapporo, Japan

H. Takigawa
Department of Urology, School of Medicine, Tokushima University, Tokushima, Japan

K. Tanaka
Institute for Enzyme Research, Tokushima University, Tokushima, Japan

M. Terada
National Cancer Centre, Chuo-ku, Tokyo, Japan

M. Togashi
Department of Urology, Hokkaido University School of Medicine, Sapporo, Japan

M. Toro-Rojas
Pathology Unit, Córdoba University Medical School and Reina Sofia University Hospital, Córdoba, Spain

T. Uchibayashi
Department of Urology, School of Medicine, Kanazawa University, Kanazawa, Japan

K. Uema
Department of Urology, School of Medicine, Tokushima University, Tokushima, Japan

P. J. Walther
Division of Urology, Duke University School of Medicine, Durham, North Carolina, USA

Y. Watabe
Department of Urology, School of Medicine, Chiba University, Chiba, Japan

O. Yoshida
Department of Urology, Faculty of Medicine, Kyoto University, Kyoto, Japan

A. Zervas
Departments of Urology and Pathology, Athens University Medical School, Athens, Greece

A. R. Zhou
Institute of Urology, Beijing Medical University, Beijing, China

V. Zolota
Departments of Urology and Pathology, Athens University Medical School, Athens, Greece

Introduction

C. A. Olsson

Progress in molecular biology can be likened to that seen in aeronautics. In a man's single lifetime, aeronautics has seen the development of manned space travel from his initial flight at Kitty Hawk. Similarly, in molecular biology progress has been prodigious since James Watson and Francis Crick determined the double helical structure of DNA in 1953.

Most of the molecular techniques employed by laboratories throughout the world have an even shorter history. Paul Berg, at Stanford University, perfected the process of DNA recombination in 1972. Stanley Cohen, also at Stanford, demonstrated the feasibility of gene cloning in 1974. Walter Gilbert and Fred Sanger, of Harvard and Cambridge Universities, respectively, shared the credit for sequencing genes in 1975. In 1977, the first human protein (growth hormone) was produced by recombinant technology. In 1980, David Botstein described the technique of restriction fragment length polymorphism as a means of locating the site of a gene on a chromosome. In 1982 Richard Palmiter and Ralph Brinster demonstrated the feasibility of transgenic technology, creating mice with extra copies of the somatastatin gene.

Progress in the field of molecular biology has developed to the point that in 1990 the world's first gene therapy was introduced. In a young girl suffering from adenosine deaminase (ADA) deficiency the girl's immune cells were extracted from her blood, transfected with copies of the gene encoding ADA, expanded in tissue culture and reinfused into the child, with the result that her immune system remains intact today. Similarly, Steven Rosenberg at the National Cancer Institute in the United States has begun a human experimentation in cancer, wherein cancer cells transfected with the gene that encodes tumor necrosis factor are reinjected into the host, with the hope that the patient's own immune system will be activated against the host's cancer.

It is, therefore, appropriate that the Société Internationale d'Urologie (SIU) sponsored a program on the molecular genetics of urological cancers at its 1991 conference. It is further appropriate that the SIU has chosen to select the subject for the preparation of this monograph. With the rather astonishing developments in molecular biology, as applied specifically to urological cancers, this monograph attempts to review the progress in this area and hopes to remain a reference source for further investigations in the future.

As chairman of the conference I would like to take the opportunity to thank all the participants. Both the conference and monograph are organized similarly. Professor Donald Coffey of Baltimore presents an article explaining the applications of molecular technology to cancer investigations in general. Following this, each of our four reporters (Professor Rolf Ackerman of Dusseldorf, Professor Geoffrey Chisholm of Edinburgh, Professor Frans DeBruyne of Nijmegen and Professor Tadao Kakizoe of Tokyo present summary statements on the progress in molecular studies of the four major urological neoplasms (cancer of the testis, kidney, prostate and bladder).

Finally, following the presentations by the four reporters, a series of articles have been chosen from both the independent communications and poster sessions that accompanied the conference. These articles were chosen because of their excellence and originality.

I wish to thank again the many individuals who were so helpful in the completion of this monograph.

1. Understanding DNA changes in urological cancers

W. B. Isaacs D. S. Coffey

Understanding the changes in DNA in urological tumours will soon provide more precise diagnostic and prognostic indicators of tumour behavior. Recently, a rational new therapeutic modality involving genetic engineering of tumour cells has evolved at the experimental level that may soon be used to assist the surgeon in eradicating minimal residual disease following radical surgery. This review provides insight into the principles involved in understanding the human genome.

THE STRUCTURE OF THE CANCER CELL

The pathologist can diagnose cancer by the abnormal structure of the cancer cell. The tumour cell is characterized by a structural instability that produces a wide variation in the observed shape and size of the cell and nucleus. The large variation in shape is termed 'pleomorphism' and is now traced to alterations in the tissue matrix system; this is composed of a residual interlocking cellular scaffolding system that forms the skeleton of the tissue and remains after extracting lipid and soluble components. This tissue structural framework system extends from the extracellular matrix through the inside of the cell and cytomatrix and connects with the central nuclear matrix that provides form to the nucleus and organizes the DNA. The cell part of the matrix system is highly dynamic and the structure is capable of undergoing changes that can produce chemomechanical movement both within a cell and to produce cell motility. The cytomatrix provides a hard-wired network of structural roadways within the cell, and by time-lapse videomicroscopy small subcellular particles can be visualized travelling backwards and forwards in their translocation throughout the cell by utilizing these intracellular networks and roadways. The cell is also capable of translocating itself through intracellular chemomechanical events that provide cell motility by utilizing contractions and extensions of these cytomatrix networks. Pathology involves observing dead or fixed cells that give only a freeze-frame picture, but when cells are observed in their viable state it is apparent that cancer cells are most dynamic and have reactivated the ability to move. This is an essential mechanism in helping them to invade adjoining tissues or to metastasize.

The cancer cell is also characterized by exhibiting a large variation in gene expression, so that within any one tumour tremendous cellular heterogeneity is expressed. This has been termed pleiotropism, and is believed to be driven in part by a genetic instability in the DNA that resembles a microevolutionary process. This tremendous biological diversity in tumour cells enables them to succeed in a competitive environment that includes the selection of cell clones in the tumour that are resistant to all forms of therapeutic modalities. Cancer cells can develop rapid resistance to all known natural and synthetic drugs, while normal cells are essentially devoid of this ability to form resistant clones. As the driving force in the development of tumour cell heterogeneity is genetic instability, it is important to determine whether this is determined by cell structure, or whether instability in the DNA itself produces the instability in structure. Cancer cells are characterized by a series of instabilities that increase with time and this is involved in the progression that is observed with time. We will briefly describe the organization of the cell with emphasis on how structure impacts on the organization of DNA. For a review of the concept, see Pienta et al (1989) and Getzenberg et al (1990).

THE STRUCTURAL ORGANIZATION OF THE NUCLEUS

The shape of the nucleus is determined by the nuclear matrix; this is the dynamic structural subcomponent of the nucleus that directs the three-dimensional organization of DNA into loop domains and provides sites for the specific control of nucleic acid intranuclear and particulate transport (Pienta et al 1991). The nuclear matrix structure is essentially devoid of histones and lipids and represents less that 15% of the mass of the intact nucleus. Primarily, the nuclear matrix serves an important role in DNA organization and in determining nuclear shape and structure. The vast amount of DNA within the nucleus is organized into many DNA loop domains that are each attached and anchored at their bases to the nuclear matrix, and this organization is maintained throughout both interphase and metaphase. These loops are 50–150 kbp long and are equivalent in size to the replicon, i.e., the amount of DNA replicated as a unit during DNA synthesis that resides between adjacent replicating forks. There are approximately 50 000 to 100 000 of these DNA loops per nucleus. The DNA loops are often supercoiled, which may in part control the chromatin structure through regulation of DNA winding and topology by topoisomerase enzymes.

The nuclear matrix also plays an important role in DNA replication. The matrix contains fixed sites for DNA synthesis, also located at the base of each loop. During DNA synthesis the loop domains are reeled down through the attached replicating complexes. The DNA replication fork, DNA polymerase α, and newly replicated DNA are all closely associated with the nuclear matrix during DNA synthesis. Therefore, the nuclear matrix is well positioned to play an important structural role in the organization and biological control of DNA during eukaryotic replication. Furthermore, when DNA viruses replicate in a mammalian cell they to are synthesized in association with the nuclear matrix of the host cell. It is easy to visualize how alteration in the nuclear matrix structures that occurs with cancer and the associated aberrant nuclear shapes could impinge on the regulation of DNA synthesis.

The nuclear matrix is also associated with transcription of the gene into messenger RNA (mRNA). Transcriptional complexes have been identified in the nuclear matrix and mRNA is transported out of the nucleus on roadways composed of the nuclear matrix. Many studies with a wide variety of genes have demonstrated that active genes are associated with the nuclear matrix while transcriptionally inactive genes are not, providing further evidence that the matrix may play an important organizing role in transcriptional functions and gene expression.

The nuclear matrix is a major site of steroid hormone receptor binding since 40–60% of all nuclear steroid receptors (oestrogens or androgens) are associated with this matrix. In addition, the nuclear acceptor for the steroid-bound receptor appears to be part of the nuclear matrix in steroid target tissues. The nuclear matrix proteins, localized to the interior of the nucleus, vary in a cell type-specific manner, suggesting that the nuclear matrix may play an important role in development and tissue organization (Getzenberg & Coffey 1990).

In cancer cells transformation proteins appear to be associated with the nucleus, and many of these appear to be involved with the matrix. For example, the nuclear matrix is reported to be one of the targets for retrovirus *myc* oncogene protein, adenovirus E1A-transforming protein, and polyoma large T antigen. It remains to be resolved how these viral proteins induce cell division, but with normal cell growth, numatrin, a nuclear matrix protein, has been associated with the induction of mitogenesis. The nuclear matrix has been shown to be altered during transformation by producing a change in protein composition. Since steroid receptors and transforming proteins such as the nuclear oncogene products affect DNA function in target cells, more insight is required into how these proteins alter the functions of the nuclear matrix and DNA organization.

THE ORGANIZATION OF DNA WITHIN THE NUCLEUS

The long length of DNA of over 2 metres is packed into a 10-micron nucleus, resulting in a condensation in DNA length of 40 000-fold. The double helix is first wrapped around an octomer of histones termed the 'nucleosome'. Six of these nucleosomes are wrapped into a circle to form a turn of solenoid that is the 30-nM filament that will make the filament of the DNA loops. The DNA loop domain defines a basic unit of higher order DNA structure which is present throughout the cell cycle in eukaryotic cells.

These loops have an average of 63 ± 14 kbp. An average loop would be large enough to contain 300 nucleosomes. If a human diploid nucleus contains 6×10^9 base pairs, there would be approximately 100 000 of these DNA loop domains within a single nucleus. In metaphase, DNA loop domains are preserved in chromosomes, with the loops wrapped radially around the central axis of the chromatid as they stack like a 'slinky' to achieve the overall chromosome length. Our analysis revealed that there would be 18 DNA loops per radial turn of the chromatid to form a 'miniband'. The miniband, or one turn around the chromosome, is equivalent to one full radial turn of 18 loops, each of 60 kbp, which is formed around the central axis of the chromatid to form minibands of approximately one million base pairs of DNA (18 × 60 kbp). The DNA loop domains present in the metaphase chromosome maintain their association with the nuclear matrix in the interphase nucleus. The telomere regions on the end of the chromosome are attached to the peripheral lamina. During mitosis, the nuclear lamina proteins under the nuclear envelope are phosphorylated and diffuse as small vesicles into the cytoplasmic area as the nuclear envelope disintegrates. The chromosomes, now free of the lamina, collapse into a condensed mitotic structure. The nuclear matrix structures at the base of the DNA loops are maintained as the core scaffolding or matrix within the centre of the chromosome. At the end of telophase, the ends of the chromosome serve as an organizing centre for the condensation of lamina proteins to reform the lamina and nuclear envelope of the nucleus.

The nuclear matrix-DNA complex is altered with the development of cancer, and this is observed grossly as a distorted nuclear shape and structure (pleomorphism). The altered matrix could alter chromatin packing, and this is believed to affect tumour cell genetic instability.

DNA INSTABILITY IN CANCER CELLS

Instability in chromosome structure occurs in many cancers. Chromosome translocations have been proposed to be a common factor in many types of human neoplasias. When large translocations occur, there is also a transfer of chromosomal banding patterns. Structural elements of the core scaffold of the chromosome and the nuclear matrix that anchor the DNA loops of the chromosome must also be transferred in the translocation process. Since sister chromatid exchanges occur at the site of DNA replication that is located on the matrix, the nuclear matrix components may be involved in these rearrangements. These types of DNA reorganization in cancer, that include gene amplification, sister chromatid exchange, and a series of different subtypes of rearrangements and deletions, have all been demonstrated in both animal and human tumours (Fig. 1.1). Each of these processes involves a change in the order of arrangement of the DNA sequence and as such has been proposed to be involved in the initiation of carcinogenesis and/or increase progression. Any of these rearrangements

TYPES	DNA ALTERATIONS
Normal	CH_3 on C: A - T - G - C - A - G - G - C - T - A ......
Hypomethylation	A - T - G - [C] - A - G - G - C - T - A ...... (Loss of Methyl)
Hypermethylation	CH_3 on both C: A - T - G - C - A - G - G - C - T - A ...... (Add Methyl)
Point mutation	A - T - G - [A] - A - G - G - C - T - A ...... (Change of Base)
Rearrangement	CH_3 on C: A - T - G - C - [C - T - A] - A - G - G ...... (Relocated)
Deletion	CH_3 on C: A - T - G - C - [A - G - G - C] - T - A ...... (Deleted)
Amplification	CH_3 on each C: A - T - [G - C - A - G - C - A] - [G - C - A] - G - G

Fig. 1.1 Examples of the six types of DNA changes associated with cancer.

which bestows a growth advantage on the cells could cause a hyperplasia or tumour formation. If a DNA rearrangement places an error within the genomic apparatus such that further genetic instability ensues, a wide variety of cells would result. This type of genetic instability may be the basis of progression with time and the ultimate formation of tumour cell heterogeneity. Elucidation of the molecular events which produce this genetic instability is critical to the understanding of cancer. It will be necessary to define the relationship between genetic instability and the alterations of cancer cell structure, which is the morphological hallmark of cancer diagnosis, in order to further our understanding of the cancer process. The concept of a dynamic tissue matrix system appears to form a basis for this understanding.

GENES AND CANCERS: ONCOGENES AND TUMOUR SUPPRESSOR GENES

Human cancer cells contain DNA sequences (oncogenes) which, when added back (transfected) into normal cells, cause neoplastic transformation. These oncogenes are found to be activated or inappropriately expressed in tumours, and about 10–30% of human tumours contain such activated oncogenes. Multiple oncogene expressions are required to produce a malignant transformation. The oncogene protein products found to be expressed from these oncogenes include nuclear proteins that activate

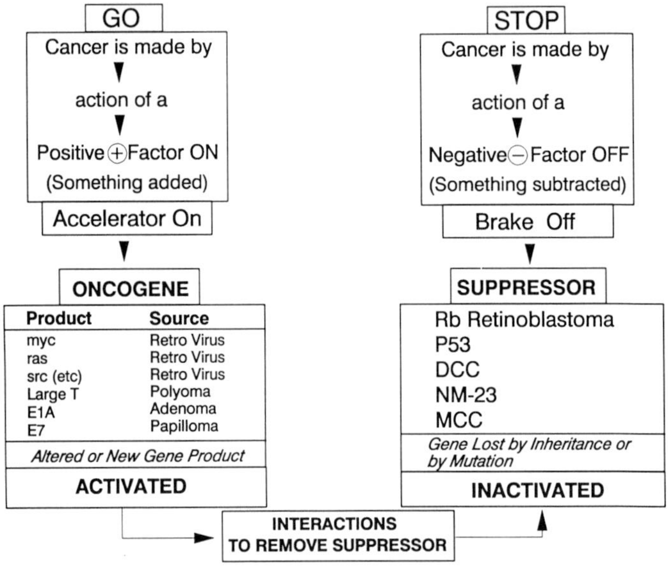

Fig. 1.2 The concept of the oncogene and suppressor gene.

other genes and are therefore serving as transcription factors, and oncogene products that enhance the cell signalling pathway by which growth factors signal through the cell to the nucleus to activate growth. Many of these oncogene products are aberrant normal products and appear to continue the stimulation of the cell and cannot be down-regulated or shut off. *Oncogenes* are seen as 'on signals' for growth in that they have to be activated and are therefore a *positive factor.* The inappropriate expression of an oncogene may be seen as analogous to an accelerator pedal being stuck to the floor causing excess growth (Fig. 2.2). The oncogenes are mutated in viruses and infections and incorporation into host DNA may be involved in cancer formation. Complications in this simple 'on signal' concept occurred when it was discovered that when normal cells are fused to cancer cells to form a new hybrid cell, they are usually demonstrated in normal phenotype. This indicated that there is something in normal cells that suppresses the expression of the tumour phenotype, a factor termed a *suppressor.* A study of these normal suppressor factors indicated that genes that produce negative factors, or brakes, exist in normal cells and suppress growth, but are not present in cancer cells. Therefore, fusing the normal cell and the cancer cell together produces a cell that applies the brakes to growth and makes the fused cell more normal. More insight was gained into how oncogenes and suppressors interact when it was discovered that some oncogene products can actually bind to the suppressor proteins and inactivate the braking system; this is one mechanism by which they release the growth inhibition on normal cells. In summary, there is an 'on' and 'off' switch similar to a brake and accelerator that have been termed 'oncogenes' and 'suppressors', respectively.

In cancer, the *inactivation of the suppressor*, with the subsequent release of the brake on growth, could occur by either mutating a gene so that it does not work as a brake (inactivation), or by *deleting* it from the chromosome. Since there are two copies of each gene (alleles) in a cell, one inherited from the mother and one from the father, it would require inactivation of both copies to fully release the brake on growth. When certain areas of chromosomes are observed to be deleted in association with cancer, it usually indicates the possibility that the other copy of the same gene is also inactivated or mutated so that both alleles are inactivated.

The series of genetic events which occur in human carcinogenesis and progression have been most extensively characterized by Bert Vogelstein at Johns Hopkins in his classic studies of colorectal cancer. The genetic alterations include hypomethylation of DNA, activation of one of the oncogenes (Ki-ras), and loss of genetic information from chromosome 17p, 18q and 5q. The identification of the tumour suppressor gene on chromosome 17p showed it to encode a protein of molecular weight 53 000, termed *p53*. The p53 protein is most commonly inactivated by allelic loss of one copy and mutation of the remaining copy of the p53 gene. In either experiment in vitro, it was demonstrated that if the mutated p53 gene in the cancer cell was replaced with a normal copy of p53 gene, it would suppress the growth of the cancer cells. Other genes on chromosomes 18p, termed DCC (deleted in colorectal cancer) and MCC (mutated in colorectal cancer), have recently been identified as suppressor genes. At present, it does not appear that any specific order of these genetic changes is required for cancer; rather, it is the accumulation of these alterations in DNA that can be correlated with disease progression. It is not yet known what sets off the genetic instability that causes these genetic changes, nor whether it is an alteration in cell structure or an alteration that occurs in some gene that increases the rate of changes or mutations in other genes. Some DNA alterations that have been implicated in causing genetic instability are changes in DNA methylation, primarily because it occurs early in carcinogenesis. Normally, only 4% of the cytosine residues within the genomic DNA are methylated on the 5′ position of cytosine. Methylated cytosines are always 5′ to the guanine residues (CG-dinucleotide). It is known that these methylation patterns of cytosine change in development and that hypermethylation of DNA is associated with gene inactivation, whereas hypomethylated genes may or may not be active. Tumour DNA is generally *hypomethylated*, but there are specific areas of hypermethylation in some genes and this may be associated with tumour suppressor gene inactivation. It is not known what regulates the abnormal pattern of methylation of cytosine that is associated with cancer.

A COMMON GENE ALTERED IN CANCER IS p53

A 53 000 molecular weight phosphoprotein (p53) is present in the nucleus of virtually all cells. The normal form of the p53 protein is present in very small amounts due to a short half-life of approximately 15 minutes. It has some paradoxical effects. Although normally acting as a suppressor or 'off signal' for cell growth, mutant forms of p53 also have the ability to act as an 'on signal' or like an oncogene. p53 is elevated in many transformed cells due to an increase in its half-life and it has the ability to cooperate with other oncogenes to transform cells. It is believed that some mutant forms of p53 can bind to the normal form of p53 to form a dimer, resulting in the loss of growth-suppressive function of the normal p53 protein. The mechanism by which p53 normally functions is unknown but it appears to bind directly to the DNA and may regulate some aspects of the cell cycle. Mutations of p53 have been found at a high frequency in human cancers of the colon, breast, lung, bladder, brain, liver and prostate. Almost all these mutations are present in exons 5–8, an evolutionary conserved region, presumably critical for p53 function. p53 has also been shown to be a target for chemical carcinogenesis producing specific sites of mutation for different carcinogens.

GENETIC CHANGES IN BLADDER CANCER

Early studies suggested that the *ras* oncogene mutation was a frequent event in bladder cancer but this later turned out to be a characteristic only of cultured bladder cancer cells and is not very common in the primary human bladder cancers. Loss of heterozygosity has been observed in chromosomes 9q, 11p and 17p (Tsai et al 1990). Both superficial and muscle-invasive bladder carcinomas show allelic loss of chromosome 9q, but the gene located in this region has not yet been identified. Muscle-invasive tumours show additional allelic loss frequency on chromosome 17p (Olumi 1990). Over 60% of these muscle-invasive tumours contain a mutated p53 allele and in over 90% of these tumours this mutation is coupled with an allelic loss in the 17p region containing the p53 gene (Sidransky et al 1991). Recently, p53 mutations have been detected in the DNA of urine sediments in untreated bladder cancer patients, providing the possibility of screening for high-risk individuals or conducting follow-ups after partial cystectomy (Sidransky et al 1991).

GENETIC CHANGES IN PROSTATE CANCER

A mutated ras oncogene in prostate cancer has been shown to be a relatively rare event occurring in less than 5% of prostate cancer samples, derived from either primary or metastatic tumours (Carter et al 1990a,b). Studies of allelic loss as well as karyotype studies have shown deletions of the long arm of chromosome 10 to be the most consistent chromosomal abnormality observed in prostate cancer, although this change is far from universal (Carter et al 1990b, Brothman et al 1990). In addition, loss of genetic material from chromosomes 8p and 16q has been reported to occur at significant frequencies in prostate cancer. At present, no candidate suppressor genes in these specific regions of the chromosomes have been identified to indicate the nature of the important genetic information lost in association with prostate cancer.

The first mutated genes in human prostate cancer have now been identified and p53 appears to be an important target (Isaacs et al 1991). Mutations of the p53 gene have been identified in both prostate cancer cell lines and in primary and metastatic deposits of prostate cancer. In addition, the growth suppressive effect of a normal p53 gene reintroduced into prostate cancer cells has been demonstrated (Isaacs et al 1991). This is equivalent to introducing a normal operating brake into the cancer cell to stop growth of the cancer. The overall frequency of p53 mutations in human prostate cancers and their role in tumour progression remain to be determined.

It has also been observed that mutations in the androgen receptor gene are associated with androgen-resistant human prostate tumours (Newmark et al 1991). It remains to be seen if this is a common pathway by which prostate cancer escapes androgen ablation.

Other candidate genes involved in prostate cancer include the retinoblastoma gene; this appears to be modified in prostate cancer but the exact frequency has not been established (Bookstein et al 1990).

Recently, it has been established that there are clear familial aspects in some forms of prostate cancer and it will be most important to study the genetic alterations that occur in these pedigrees (Steinberg et al 1990).

GENETIC CHANGES IN RENAL CELL CANCER

Loss of heterozygosity and deletions in chromosome 3p, trisomy 7, and a nonreciprocal translocation in chromosomes 5 and 14, have been implicated as the potential primary event in the development of renal cancers (Weaver et al 1989). Close attention has been focused on chromosome 3, where the loss in the short arm can occur by interstitial deletion, nonreciprocal chromosome translocation or the loss of the entire chromosome. A fragile site occurs at 3p14 and a loss of heterozygosity is most readily detected at 3p21 at a locus defined as DNF15S2 (Zbar et al 1987, Bergerheim et al 1989).

Examples of familial renal cancer include von Hippel-Lindau disease (VHL), an autosomal dominant syndrome with a 30% incidence of associated renal cell cancer at autopsy. The gene for VHL has been mapped by linkage analysis to chromosome 3p25 (Seizinger et al 1988). At present, great efforts are underway to define the chromosomal abnormalities occurring on chromosomes 3, 5, 7 and 14 that are associated with or involved in the causality of renal cell cancer.

GENETICALLY ENGINEERED TUMOUR VACCINES

Pardoll and associates have pioneered a new method of immunological therapy for cancer that appears to have great promise (Fearon et al 1988, Golumbek et al 1991). Steven Rosenberg, of the National Cancer Institute team, had earlier pioneered the use of cytokines, such as interleukins, as biological therapy to control cancer growth (Rosenberg et al 1988a,b). Cytokines are growth factors and modulators of the immune system that are released by cells to regulate the immune response. In the earlier studies, interleukin 2 (IL-2) was used as a drug by injection but was soon found to be too toxic in relation to its therapeutic advantage. Attention soon turned to isolating tumour-infiltrating lymphocytes (TIL), expanding them by growing them in culture, and then injecting the increased number of TIL back into the host in a form of cell therapy, in the hope that the stimulated lymphocytes would immunologically attack the cancer cells. This is still under investigation and further development will obviously be needed to bring it to its clinical usefulness.

Fearon and colleagues (Fearon et al 1990) decided to take an entirely different approach. Their rationale was to remove a few tumour cells, and modify them by genetic manipulation so that the tumour cells themselves would express antigens or cytokines that would enhance nearby immune cells to increase the immune system's ability to then attack the other tumour cells in patients which had not been so modified. This approach was accomplished when Pardoll transfected isolated host tumour cells with expression vectors containing various interleukin genes that were in proximity to strong promoters which allowed the strong overexpression of interleukins by the tumour cell. When lymphocytes approach these tumour cells, they encounter a very high local concentration of interleukin from the overexpressed gene in the tumour; the neighbouring lymphocytes are therefore stimulated to divide and expand in number and to recognize and attack tumour cells in the host. This technique has been studied in renal cell cancer and in prostate cancer (Moody et al 1991) in animal model systems and shown to immunologically protect these animals against subsequent challenges by unmodified tumour cells. More recently, it has been shown by Pardoll's laboratory that established tumours can also be treated with such cell therapy. Pardoll's technique is now being actively pursued by the National Cancer Institute and other laboratories, and it is hoped that it will soon be available for human application. At present this approach appears to be most effective against low tumour volume and minimal disease. It would therefore be most beneficial to apply cell therapy after radical surgery in bulk removal of primary and metastatic lesions.

It is apparent that a clearer understanding of genetic changes in cancer will be essential to diagnose and to counsel the patient. It is hoped that genetic engineering of tumour cells, as described above for cell therapy, will help to control these devastating urological cancers. It is visualized that significant progress will be made by combining early diagnosis leading to radical surgery to eliminate bulk tumour burden, with cell therapeutic approaches to eradicate micrometastatic and minimal residual cancer. These powerful new techniques will undoubtedly have a profound impact on the future of urology.

REFERENCES

Bergerheim U, Nordenskjold M, Collins V P 1989 Deletion mapping in human renal cell carcinoma. Cancer Res 49: 1390–1396

Bookstein R, Shew J, Chen P et al 1990 Suppression of tumorigenicity of human prostate carcinoma cells by replacing a mutated Rb gene. Science 247: 712–715

Brothman A, Peehl D, Patel A et al 1990 Frequency and pattern of karyotypic abnormalities in human prostatic cancer. Cancer Res 50: 3795–3803

Carter B S, Epstein J I, Isaacs W B 1990a *ras* gene mutations in human prostate cancer. Cancer Res 50: 6830–6832

Carter B S, Ewing C M, Ward W S et al 1990b Allelic loss on chromosomes 10q and 16q in human prostate cancer. Proc Nat Acad Sci USA 87: 8751–8755

Fearon E R, Itaya T, Hunt B et al 1988 Induction in a murine tumor of immunogenic tumor variants by transfection with a foreign gene. Cancer Res 48: 2975–2980

Fearon E R, Pardoll D M, Itaya T et al 1990 Interleukin–2 production by tumor cells bypasses T helper function in the generation of an antitumor response. Cell 60: 397–403

Getzenberg R H, Coffey D S 1990 Tissue specificity of the hormonal response in sex accessory tissues is associated with nuclear matrix and protein patterns. Mol Endocrinol 4: 1336–1342

Getzenberg R H, Pienta K J, Coffey D S 1990 Tissue matrix: cell dynamics and hormone action. Endocr Rev 11: 399–417

Golumbek F M, Lazenby A J, Levitsky H I et al 1991 Tumors engineered to secrete interleukin-4 generate antigen-specific T cell-mediated immunity. Science 254: 713–716

Isaacs W B, Carter B S, Ewing C M 1991 Wild-type p53 suppresses growth of human prostate cancer cells containing mutant p53 alleles. Cancer Res 51: 4716–4720

Moody D B, Ewing C M, Isaacs W B 1991 Lymphokine-transfected prostate cancer cells generate an anti-tumor effect in vivo. J Urol 145: 293A

Newmark J R, Hardy D O, Carter B A et al 1991 Androgen receptor gene mutations in androgen independent human prostate cancer tissue and cell lines. J Urol 145: 349A

Olumi A F, Tsai Y C, Nichols P W et al 1990 Allelic loss of chromosome 17p distinguishes high grade from low grade transitional cell carcinoma of the bladder. Cancer Res 50: 7081–7083

Pienta K J, Partin A W, Coffey D S 1989 Cancer as a disease of DNA organization and dynamic cell structure. Cancer Res 49: 2526–2532

Pienta K J, Getzenberg R H, Coffey D S 1991 Cell structure and DNA organization. Critical Reviews in Eukaryotic Gene Expression 1: 335–385

Rosenberg S A, Packard B S, Aebersold P M et al 1988a Use of tumor-infiltrating lymphocytes and interleukin–2 in the immunotherapy of patients with metastatic melanoma. A preliminary report. New Eng J Med 319: 1676–1680

Rosenberg S A, Schwarz S L, Spiess P J 1988b Combination immunotherapy for cancer: synergistic antitum or interactions of interleukin-2, alfa interferon, and tumor-infiltrating lymphocytes. J Natl Cancer Inst 80: 1393–1397

Seizinger B R, Rouleau G A, Ozelius L J et al 1988 von Hippel-Lindau disease maps to the region of chromosome 3 associated with renal cell carcinoma. Nature 332: 268–269

Sidransky D, von Eschenbach A C, Tsai T C et al 1991 Identification of p53 gene mutations in bladder cancers and urine samples. Science 252: 706–709

Steinberg G D, Carter B S, Beaty T H et al 1990 Family history and the risk of prostate cancer. Prostate 17: 337–347

Tsai Y, Nichols P, Hiti A et al 1990 Allelic losses of chromosomes 9, 11 and 17 in human bladder cancer. Cancer Res 50: 44–47
Weaver D J, Michalski K, Miles J H 1989 Cytogenetics of bilateral renal cell carcinoma. J Urol 142: 697–700
Zbar B, Brauch H, Talmadge C et al 1987 Loss of alleles of loci on the short arm of chromosome 3 in renal cell carcinoma. Nature 327: 721–724

2. Oncogenes and molecular genetics of renal tumours

G. D. Chisholm

One of the characteristic features of cancer cells is that the normal growth control mechanisms are defective. We know something of the factors that control cell division though this knowledge is far from complete. The process of contact inhibition regulates the development of new cells when they are needed (Folkman & Moscona 1978). Other important processes that are needed for cell growth include a positional requirement (French et al 1976) and the role of minute amounts of growth factors which act systemically as well as locally in cell-to-cell interaction (Real et al 1986).

Much of our understanding of the regulation of normal growth has come from the study of viruses and their interaction to produce cancer. Many RNA tumour viruses (retroviruses) are known to exist, and study of these has been important because of their ability to transform some normal cells into malignant cells. One of the mechanisms for this malignant transformation involves the effect of oncogenes – genetic segments capable of this transformation. Thus, oncogenes, whether generated by quantitative or qualitative alterations of normal cellular genes, contribute to the process of malignant transformation. Oncogenes do not, however, explain the hereditary component of many tumours. Studies of patients in cancer families or those individuals with multiple tumours suggest that there is an inherited loss of genetic elements of tumour suppressor genes or anti-oncogenes (Hansen & Cavenee 1987; see Table 2.1).

The hallmark for this existence of a tumour suppressor gene or anti-oncogene is the demonstration of nonrandom DNA loss in neoplastic tissue when compared with normal tissue DNA in the same patient (Ponder 1988). Several genito-urinary tumours have also exhibited this nonrandom loss of DNA on various chromosomes. This communication refers to findings related only to kidney tumours.

RENAL CELL CANCER

This tumour is the most common adult malignancy; it usually occurs in the sporadic form but familial renal cell cancers have been reported. Both forms are associated with a translocation of the short arm on chromosome 3. Southern blot analysis of this region in sporadic cases demonstrated loss of

Table 2.1 Comparison of oncogenes and anti-oncogenes (de Wolf 1991).

	Oncogenes	Anti-oncogenes
Mechanisms	Activation of a proto-oncogene	Deletion of a normally suppressed gene
Hereditary	No	Sometimes
Host genetics	Sporadic	Sporadic/hereditary
Cell genetics	Dominant	Recessive

somatic DNA on chromosome 3 in a high percentage of tumours examined (Kovacs et al 1988, Zbar et al 1987). It appears that defects distal on the short arm of chromosome 3 are fundamental to the development of renal cell carcinoma. There is a high frequency of chromosomal breakage at 3p13–14 site (Kovacs et al 1987a).

The break point was detected using restriction fragment length polymorphism analysis (Zbar et al 1987, Kovacs et al 1988, Van der Hout et al 1988).

Similar deletions have been described in several lung carcinomas, particularly small cell cancer, breast cancer and uterine cancer, thus supporting the theory that loss of activity of a vital control gene may contribute to carcinogenesis in many tissue types (de Riese et al 1991).

Other less common abnormalities include trisomy for the region 5q22–qter and the deletion of 14q22–qter (Kovacs & Frisch 1989). Rukstalis & de Wolf (1990) have shown evidence of DNA loss on the short arm of chromosome 6.

Cytogenetic and molecular studies in sporadic renal cell carcinoma have consistently demonstrated chromosome 3p rearrangements. Recently, Shimizu et al (1990) reported that the introduction of a normal chromosome 3p modulated the tumorigenicity of a human renal cell carcinoma cell line. In molecular genetic studies of sporadic renal cell carcinoma, the most frequent change is allele loss from chromosome 3p21. This includes the region in which the Von Hippel-Lindau disease gene has been localized (3p25–26) but the region of the 3;8 translocation breakpoint (3p14) is not always involved. The data suggest that at least two loci on chromosome 3p are involved in the pathogenesis of non-familial renal cell carcinoma. One locus is situated distally and may be the Von Hippel-Lindau disease gene itself; the other is more proximal (3p13–21) and may be the site of the translocation breakpoints at 3p13 or 3p14. Kovacs & Hoene (1988) have reported a nonfamilial renal cancer in a patient with a constitutional 3;12 translocation with a break point at 3q13.2 in whom the derivative chromosome containing 3p was lost from the tumour cells. Thus renal cell carcinoma seems to be similar to Wilms' tumour in that multiple loci are involved. Further studies of constitutional chromosome 3 rearrangements will be necessary to clarify the significance of these translocations.

Thus, molecular genetic studies of chromosome 3 indicate that this is the marker chromosome for renal cell carcinoma (de Riese et al 1991).

FAMILIAL RENAL CELL CARCINOMA

Familial renal cancers are characterized by their early age at onset compared to sporadic cases, frequent bilaterality and multicentricity. The mean age at diagnosis in familial cases is about 45 years compared with 60 years for sporadic cases. There are two main groups of renal cell carcinoma:

a. those that occur as part of the von Hippel-Lindau (VHL) disease
b. those that occur without additional features (Maher & Yates 1991).

VON HIPPEL-LINDAU DISEASE

This is the most frequent cause of inherited renal cell carcinoma, and subclinical evidence of VHL disease should be sought in all cases of inherited or multiple renal cell carcinoma. The syndrome is autosomal dominant and has a heterozygote prevalence of 1:50000 persons. The characteristic features of VHL disease are retinal, cerebellar and spinal haemangioblastomas, renal carcinoma, phaeochromocytoma and renal, pancreatic and epididymal cysts. Most patients with VHL disease present before the age of 40 years and almost all gene carriers can be identified by the age of 60 if appropriate screening is performed (Maher & Yates 1991). Although renal carcinoma is the presenting feature in only 10% of patients with VHL disease, the risk of developing renal cell carcinoma rises progressively from the age of 20 and is 70% by the age of 60 years.

FAMILIAL RENAL CELL CARCINOMA WITHOUT ADDITIONAL FEATURES

The literature contains 23 reports of 105 patients with familial renal cell carcinoma. The mean age at diagnosis of these patients is about 45 years. The most likely mode of inheritance is autosomal dominant with age-dependent penetrants, vertical transmission being observed in 17 of 29 families available for analysis.

In 1979 Cohen et al reported the cytogenetic analysis of 10 members of a family predisposed to renal cell carcinoma and showed a constitutional reciprocal translocation of chromosomes 3 and 8. Similar studies since then have shown frequent aberrations of chromosome 3 including the translocation and deletion of chromosome bands, with the break point in the region of 3p11.2–p13 (Kovacs et al 1987a). Other less common abnormalities include trisomy for the region 5q22–qter and the deletion of 14q22–qter

(Kovacs & Frisch 1989). The translocation of chromosome 8q24.13–qter to the short arm of chromosome 3 in familial RCC has been shown to involve the translocation of c-myc (Drabkin et al 1985). It is suggested that the expression of an altered c-myc protein may be involved in a carcinogenesis of renal cell carcinoma, possibly stimulating cellular proliferation. Several studies have demonstrated the enhanced expression of c-myc in renal cell carcinoma (Karthaus et al 1986, Yao et al 1988).

Recent research on the molecular genetics of human inherited renal cell carcinoma continues to show that it is the genes on the short arm of chromosome 3 that are implicated in the pathogenesis of familial and nonfamilial renal cell cancer (Kovacs 1989). Reports of cytogenetic deletions and allele loss in VHL disease tumours are compatible with the VHL gene functioning as a recessive tumour suppressor gene.

The expression of the oncogene c-Ha-ras has been found in renal cell carcinoma with point mutations within codons 12 and 61 (Karthaus et al 1986, Fujita et al 1988). The role of c-ras genes in malignant transformation is not certain but they appear to play a role in this multistep process (Fujita et al 1988). Other in-vitro studies have demonstrated the ability of oncogenic c-myc and c-ras products to act in the induction of carcinogenesis (Yao et al 1988). However, Nanus et al (1990) have recently demonstrated that ras oncogenes do not play a major role in the initiation, maintenance or metastasis of renal carcinomas. The proto-oncogene c-erbB1 has been found to exhibit enhanced expression in renal cell carcinomas when compared to normal kidney tissue from the same patient (Yao et al 1988). The occurrence of c-erbB2 proto-oncogene has also been reported in renal cancer (Yokota et al 1986). Apparently, many of the tumours with increased c-erbB1 expression also exhibit increases in c-myc mRNA levels. It is suggested that elevated levels of c-myc may represent a final common pathway for the stimulation of abnormal cellular proliferation in human renal cell carcinoma.

Patients with familial or multicentric renal carcinomas should be investigated for subclinical evidence of Von Hippel-Lindau disease and for chromosome 3 rearrangements. Relatives at risk should be identified and offered appropriate screening investigations. As the risk of recurrent tumours is high, all of these patients should receive lifelong follow-up (Maher & Yates 1991).

RENAL ONCOCYTOMAS

Renal oncocytomas are a distinct form of renal tumour with a characteristic morphology. These tumours are considered to be benign but Leiber et al (1981) have identified a subgroup that occasionally metastasize. The occurrence of bilateral renal oncocytomas and rare families with renal oncocytomas has suggested that genetic factors may play a role (Zhang et al 1985) and attempts have been made to identify these abnormalities. Flow cytometric studies of 42 renal oncocytomas showed that 50% were diploid, 39% were tetraploid and 11% aneuploid (Rainwater et al 1986). Cytogenetic studies have not detected a common karyotypic change (Kovacs et al 1987b). Recent cytogenetic studies and two renal oncocytomas have shown a mosaic pattern of cells with normal and abnormal karyotypes. No recurrent chromosomal aberration and no rearrangement of chromosome 3p was found. However, a characteristic restriction pattern of mitochondrial DNA was detected in these oncocytomas (Kovacs et al 1989). This finding appears to support the hypothesis that specific alterations in mitochondrial DNA may be responsible for the development of this peculiar type of tumour.

Further attempts have been made to determine whether these tumours share the genetic changes characteristic of renal carcinomas. Brauch et al (1990) analyzed chromosome 3p in five renal oncocytomas and found no chromosome changes, suggesting that a renal oncocytoma is a genetically different form of renal tumour from renal cell carcinoma.

WILMS' TUMOUR (NEPHROBLASTOMA)

Wilms' tumour or nephroblastoma is one of the commonest solid paediatric malignant tumours, accounting for 8% of childhood cancers. It affects approximately 1 in 10000 children and occurs to much the same extent worldwide. It demonstrates both an inherited and a sporadic pattern. Wilms' tumour is now a classic example of a tumour occurring in a developmental rather than an adult gene and the suppressor gene has now been isolated (Pritchard-Jones & Hastie 1990).

Wilms' tumour, like retinoblastoma, is made up of incompletely differentiated tissue. It may occur unilaterally or bilaterally with single or multiple foci. The inheritance of a predisposing gene or the presence of a specific constitutional chromosomal deletion is associated with multiple tumours and earlier onset; sporadic tumours tend to be singular and are diagnosed later in life.

The first congenital abnormality to be associated with Wilms' tumour was sporadic aniridia (Miller et al 1964). Such patients often have abnormalities in the urinary tract as well as mental retardation.

Three other recognized syndromes carry an increased risk of Wilms' tumour:

a. *Beckwith-Wiedemann syndrome*, characterized by prenatal and postnatal gigantism as well as a spectrum of other abnormalities (Smith 1988). These children have an increased risk for developing hepatoblastoma and rhabdomyosarcoma as well as Wilms' tumour. Each of these tumours has also been found to have deletions at chromosome 11p13. This parallels the finding in retinoblastoma and renal cell carcinoma, where the inactivation of an important control gene appears to be central to the development of tumours in several tissue types.

b. *Perlman syndrome*, characterized by fetal gigantism, bilateral nephromegaly with nephroblastomatosis, cryptorchidism in males and various other abnormalities (Greenberg et al 1988).
c. *Drash syndrome*, characterized by the triad of male pseudohermaphroditism, renal insufficiency and Wilms' tumour (Drash et al 1970). These children are at risk not only of Wilms' tumour but also of gonadal tumours.

Most of the children with Wilms' tumour and aniridia have a cytogenetically visible deletion in the short arm of chromosome 11 (11p13) (Riccardi et al 1978, Francke et al 1979). Aniridia is a fully penetrant abnormality, but Wilms' tumour develops in only 30–50% of patients. The male: female ratio is 2:1 and more than half of these XY patients will have associated genital abnormalities.

There is now karyotypic evidence of a specific deletion of band p13 on chromosome 11 in both sporadic and inherited forms of the disease; this has suggested the existence of an important tumour suppressor gene at this location (Slater 1986). Following the successful cloning of the retinoblastoma gene, and using the same general strategy, genes have been cloned for Duchenne muscular dystrophy, X-linked chronic granulomatous disease and retinoblastoma. In 1990, Gessler et al reported that they have now isolated a candidate gene for Wilms' tumour located on band p13 of chromosome 11. The importance of genes on chromosome 11 had been previously emphasized by Weissman et al (1987). The ability of a Wilms' tumour cell line to induce tumours in nude mice when injected subcutaneously, was completely suppressed by the introduction of a normal human chromosome 11. (Weissman et al 1987). The recently cloned Wilms' tumour gene encodes a putative transcription factor which is likely to activate or repress the expression of other genes in kidney development (Pritchard-Jones & Hastie 1990).

Subsequent molecular analysis of nephroblastomas has indicated that about 50% show a loss of heterozygosity at 11p loci. These findings suggest that the mutation of the 11p allele and subsequent initiation or loss of the normal homologous allele are necessary for malignant transformation (Dao et al 1987, Koufos et al 1984). This would be in line with the two-hit model of Knudson & Strong (1972). However, there are still inconsistencies: Huff et al (1988) have shown a lack of linkage of familial nephroblastomas to band 11p13. Also, several epidemiological studies have indicated an increased risk if parents are exposed to certain occupational hazards (Hicks et al 1984, Bunin et al 1989).

Although the cytogenetic and molecular genetic findings have revealed important abnormalities, these abnormalities occur only in a certain proportion of tumour types. It remains to be established whether the chromosomal aberrations or the molecular genetic alterations are indeed important for the initiation of malignant transformation, or represent secondary changes occurring during neoplastic development and progression (Bannasch & Zerban 1990).

REFERENCES

Bannasch P, Zerban H 1990 Animal models and renal carcinogenesis. In: Eble J N (ed) Tumors and tumor-like conditions of the kidneys and ureters. Churchill Livingstone, Edinburgh. pp 1–34

Brauch H, Tory K, Lineham W M et al 1990 Molecular analysis of the short arm of chromosome 3 in five renal oncocytomas. J Urol 143: 622–624

Bunin G R, Nass C C, Kramer S et al 1989 Parental occupation and Wilms' tumor: results of a case-control study. Cancer Res 49: 725–729

Cohen A J, Li F P, Berg S et al 1979 Hereditary renal cell carcinoma associated with a chromosome translocation. N Engl J Med 301: 592–595

Dao D D, Schroeder W T, Chao L-Y et al 1987 Genetic mechanisms of tumor-specific loss of 11p DNA sequences in Wilms' tumor. Am J Hum Genet 41: 202–217

de Riese W, Allhof E, Werner M et al 1991 Proliferative behaviour and cytogenetic changes in human renal cell carcinoma. World Journal of Urology 9: 79–85

de Wolf W C 1991 Malignancy: underlying concepts of etiology. National history and treatment. In: Gillenwater J Y, Grayhack J T, Howards S S et al (eds) Adult and pediatric urology, 2nd edn. Mosby Year Book, St Louis. pp 373–402

Drabkin H A, Bradley C, Hart I et al 1985 Translocation of c-myc in the hereditary renal cell carcinoma associated with a t(3;8) (p14.2;q24.13) chromosomal translocation. Proc Nat Acad Sci USA 82: 6980–6984

Drash A, Sherman F, Hartmann W H et al 1970 A syndrome of pseudohermaphroditism, Wilms' tumor, hypertension and degenerative renal disease. J Pediatr 76: 585–593

Folkman J, Moscona A 1978 The role of cell shape in growth control. Nature 273: 345–349

Francke U, Holmes L B, Atkins L et al 1979 Aniridia–Wilms' tumour associated: and evidence for specific deletion of 11p13. Cytogenet Cell Genet 24: 185–192

French V, Bryant P J, Bryant S V 1976 Pattern regulation in eprimorphic fields. Science 193: 969–981

Fujita J, Kraus M A, Onone H et al 1988 Activated H-ras oncogenes in human kidney tumors. Cancer Res 48: 5251–5255

Gessler M, Poustka A, Cavenee W et al 1990 Homozygous deletion in Wilms' tumour of a zinc-finger gene identified by chromosome jumping. Nature 343: 774–778

Greenberg F, Copeland K, Gresik M V 1988 Expanding the spectrum of the Perlman syndrome. Am J Med Genet 29: 773–776

Hansen M F, Cavenee W K 1987 Genetics of cancer predisposition. Cancer Res 47: 5518–5527

Hicks N, Zack M, Caldwell C G et al 1984 Childhood cancer and occupational radiation exposure in parents. Cancer 53: 1637–1643

Huff V, Compton D A, Chao L-Y et al 1988 Lack of lineage of familial Wilms' tumour to chromosomal band 11p13. Nature 336: 377–378

Karthaus H F M, Schalken J A, Feitz W F J et al 1986 Expression of the human *fes* cellular oncogene in renal cell tumors. Urol Res 14: 123–127

Knudson A G, Strong L C 1972 Mutation and cancer: a model for Wilms' tumor of the kidney. J Natl Cancer Inst 48: 313–324

Koufos A, Hansen M F, Lampkin P C et al 1984 Loss of alleles at loci on human chromosome 11 during genesis of Wilms' tumour. Nature 309: 170–172

Kovacs G, Szucs S, de Riese W et al 1987a Specific chromosome aberration in human renal carcinoma. Int J Cancer 40: 171–178

Kovacs G, Szucs S, Eichmer W et al 1987b Renal oncocytoma: a genetic and morphologic study. Cancer 59: 2071–20

Kovacs G, Erlandson R, Bozdog F et al 1988 Consistent chromosome 3p deletion and loss of heterozygosity in renal cell carcinoma. Proc Natl Acad Sci USA 85: 1571–15

Kovacs G, Hoene E 1988 Loss of der(3) in renal cell carcinoma cells of a patient with constitutional t(3;12). Hum Genet 78: 148–150

Kovacs G 1989 Papillary renal cell carcinoma. A morphologic and cytogenic study of 11 cases. Am J Pathol 134: 27–34

Kovacs G, Frisch S 1989 Clonal chromosome abnormalities in tumor cells from patients with sporadic renal cell carcinomas. Cancer Res 49: 651–659

Kovacs G, Welter C, Wilkins L et al 1989 Renal oncocytoma. A phenotypic and genotypic entity of renal parenchymal tumors. Am J Pathol 134: 967–969

Lieber M M, Tomera K M, Farran G M 1981 Renal oncocytoma. J Urol 125: 481–485

Maher E R, Yates J R W 1991 Familial renal cell carcinoma: clinical and molecular genetic aspects. Br J Cancer 63: 176–179

Miller R W, Fraumeni J F, Manning M D 1964 Association of Wilms' tumour with aniridia, hemihypertrophy and other congenital abnormalities. N Engl J Med 207: 922–927

Nanus D M, Mentle I R, Motzer R J et al 1990 Infrequent ras oncogene point mutations in renal cell carcinoma. J Urol 143: 175–178

Ponder B 1988 Gene losses in human tumours. Nature 335: 400–402

Pritchard-Jones K, Hastie N D 1990 Wilms' tumour as a paradigm for the relationship of cancer to development. Cancer Surv 9: 555–578

Rainwater L M, Farrow G M, Hay I D et al 1986 Oncocytic tumours of the salivary gland, kidney and thyroid: nuclear DNA patterns studied by flow cytometry. Br J Cancer 53: 799–804

Real F X, Rettig W J, Chesa P G et al 1986 Expression of epidermal growth factor receptor in human cultured cells and tissues: relationship to cell lineage and stage of differentiation. Cancer Res 46: 4726–4731

Riccardi V M, Sujansky E, Smith A C et al 1978 Chromosomal imbalance in the aniridia–Wilms' tumor association: 11p interstitial deletion. Pediatrics 61: 604–610

Rukstalis D B, de Wolf W C 1990 Oncogenes and antioncogenes in genitourinary malignancies. In: Lytton B (ed) Advances in Urology, vol 3 Year Book Medical Publishers, Chicago. pp 71–89

Shimizu M, Yokota J, Mori N et al 1990 Introduction of normal chromosome 3p modulates the tumorigenicity of a human renal cell carcinoma cell line YCR. Oncogene 5: 185–194

Slater RM 1986 The cytogenesis of Wilms' tumor. Cancer Genet Cytogenet 19: 37–41

Smith D W 1988 Beckwith-Wiedemann syndrome. In: Jones K L (ed) Smiths recognisable patterns of human malformation, 4th edn. W B Saunders, Philadelphia. pp 136–139

van der Hout A H, Kok K, van den Berg A et al 1988 Direct molecular analysis of a deletion of 3p in tumors from patients with sporadic renal cell carcinoma. Cancer Genet Cytogenet 32: 281–285

Weissman B E, Saxon P J, Pasquale S R et al 1987 Introduction of a normal human chromosome 11 into a Wilms' tumor cell line controls its tumorigenic expression. Science 236: 175–180

Yao M, Shuin T, Misaki H et al 1988 Enhanced expression of c-myc and epidermal growth factor receptor (c-erbB-1) genes in primary human renal cancer. Cancer Res 48: 6753–6757

Yokota J, Yamamoto T, Toyoshima K et al 1986 Amplification of c-erbB-2 oncogene in human adenocarcinomas in vivo. Lancet i: 765–766

Zbar B, Brauch H, Talmadge C et al 1987 Loss of alleles of loci on the short arm of chromosome 3 in renal cell carcinoma. Nature 327: 721–724

Zhang G, Monda L, Wasserman N F et al 1985 Bilateral renal oncocytoma: report of two cases and review of the literature. J Urol 133: 84–86

3. Oncogenes and molecular genetics of bladder cancer

T. Kakizoe K. Fujimoto M. Terada

INTRODUCTION

Transitional cell carcinoma (TCC) accounts for about 90–95% of human bladder cancer except bilharzial bladder cancer. This review will therefore primarily concentrate on TCC. The basic pattern of human bladder cancer is characterized by papillary superficial and nonpapillary (nodular) invasive tumours (Droller 1986, Kakizoe et al 1984). The former has papillary growth, usually develops in multiples, frequently features subsequent new tumour development in the bladder (recurrence) after transurethral resection (TUR), but generally has a good prognosis. The latter, on the other hand, has a nodular growth, a tendency to develop solitarily, definitely invades the muscular layer of the bladder, and consequently has a bad prognosis even when treated by radical cystectomy.

Approximately 10–20% of papillary superficial bladder cancer is reported to change to nodular invasive cancer in its natural course (Green et al 1973, Heney et al 1983, Birch & Harland 1989) and prediction of so-called 'malignant progression' is one of the serious clinical problems in the management of bladder cancer. The aforementioned clinicobiological characteristics are mutually interrelated, and our attention in this review will be focused on the differences or similarities between papillary superficial and nodular invasive bladder cancers in terms of oncogenes, suppressor genes and molecular genetics.

STEP-WISE PROGRESSION OF BLADDER CANCER

The greater number of papillary superficial bladder cancers retain their papillary superficial nature, although there is frequent recurrence (Lam & Torti 1991). About 10–20% of papillary superficial cancers change to nodular invasive cancers while repeating recurrence and this is particularly true for G3 pT1 bladder cancer (Pagano F et al 1987). Although initial tumours have a papillary growth pattern, 30–50% of G3 pT1 bladder cancers subsequently change to nodular invasive cancers (Jakse et al 1987, Abel et al 1988). At the time of first diagnosis, on the other hand, nodular invasive cancer occasionally has microscopic residual patterns of papillary growth in the tumour (Kakizoe et al 1988). This gradual shift from papillary superficial to nodular invasive cancer also has a close correlation with the grade of cancer cells. In general, papillary superficial cancers are composed of grade 1–2 cells, while nodular invasive cancers are composed of grade 2–3 cells. The grade of a tumour therefore has an association with the tumour morphology, stage and biological aggressiveness (Droller 1986).

Carcinoma in situ (CIS) of the bladder exhibits a similar growth pattern. Some CIS are composed of relatively low-grade cancer cells, and this type is often difficult to differentiate from moderate to severe dysplasia (Friedell et al 1986). It exhibits a tendency to become papillary in the direction of the bladder lumen. About half of high-grade CIS demonstrate submucosal invasion, being almost clinically separate from true CIS. Thus, if we carefully examine the clinical course and histology of bladder cancer, we can trace the step-wise shift from low-grade papillary superficial bladder cancer to high-grade nodular invasive cancer.

CYTOGENETIC MARKERS TO PREDICT PROGRESSION

Bladder cancer is a heterogeneous disease, and prediction of the possibility of progression at the time of treatment of the original tumour has been an important clinical task. In order to gain some perception of this problem, karyotyping of fresh tissue using direct techniques or short-term culture is helpful. Early studies concentrated on defining the modal number of chromosomes, the detection of aneuploidy, and the identification of marker chromosomes. Lamb (1967), using direct preparations involving 30 bladder cancers, correlated karyotypes with stage and grade. An increase in modal number of chromosomes, and an increase in structurally abnormal chromosomes were associated with loss of differentiation. All noninvasive tumours were peridiploid, while only 9% of invasive tumours were peridiploid. Spooner & Cooper (1972) correlated ploidy with grade and found that 100% of well-differentiated and moderately well-differentiated tumours were peridiploid, as compared with only 20% of poorly differentiated tumours. These authors observed that polyploidy was a common phenomenon in tumour progression, and may have resulted from successive acquisition of chromosomes, fusion of nuclei, or endoreduplications (Lerner et al 1991).

Summers et al (1981) reported on 65 patients with Ta and T1 tumours of grades 1 and 2 who were followed over 10 years. Only 2 of 20 Ta tumours without marker chromosomes recurred, but none progressed and the recurrent tumours remained marker-free. Eighteen Ta tumours with positive markers recurred, resulting in one cancer death. The 25 T1 tumours were all marker-positive; 80% of them recurred, and 12 cancer deaths occurred in a period ranging from 3 months to 6 years. The predictive value of marker chromosomes has been examined by a number of other investigators (Sandberg 1977, Milasin et al 1987). The application of flow cytometry (FCM) in bladder cancer has been extensively studied. Tumour ploidy as determined by FCM is useful in detecting recurrence (Murphy et al 1986).

MOLECULAR BIOLOGY OF BLADDER CANCER

The first example of a point mutation in a human tumour was identified in a bladder carcinoma cell line. The genetic change that leads to the activation of the cellular proto-oncogene in T24 or EJ human bladder carcinoma cells was shown to be a single point mutation of guanosine into thymidine in c-Ha-ras. This substitution resulted in the incorporation of valine instead of glycine as the twelfth amino acid residue of the c-Ha-ras-encoded p21 protein (Tabin et al 1982, Reddy et al 1982). Similar mutations in c-Ha-ras or c-Ki-ras, however, have been found in only approximately 10% of the primary human bladder cancers subsequently examined (Feinberg et al 1983, Fujita et al 1985).

The cytogenetic findings as presented in the previous section have been confirmed and extended by restriction fragment length polymorphism (RFLP) analysis. This analysis revealed frequent losses of chromosomal arms 9q, 11p, and 17p in both papillary and nodular human bladder carcinomas (Fearon et al 1985, Tsai et al 1990). In a follow-up study by Olumi et al (1990), both low-grade Ta and high-grade Ta–T4 bladder cancers were examined, and it was observed that loss of heterozygosity on chromosome 9q was independent of grade and occurred in all stages of bladder cancer. On the other hand, allelic losses of chromosome 11p (39%) and 17p (65%) were observed in only high-grade tumours, thus suggesting that loss of a tumour suppressor gene on chromosome 9q may be a primary event in the evolution of bladder cancer. These suppressor genes exert a negative regulatory effect on cancer cell growth, and when they are inactivated by mutation or deletion, the cell acquires a growth advantage comparable to that of other cells, and the neoplastic process progresses. Sidransky et al (1991) reported chromosome 17p deletions in bladder cancers reflecting underlying mutations in the p53 suppressor gene. Of 18 invasive bladder cancers evaluated, 11 (61%) had genetic alterations of p53, including 10 point mutations resulting in single amino acid substitutions, and one 24–base pair deletion.

We are also interested in mutations of the p53 suppressor gene. We investigated the structural alterations of the p53 gene to elucidate the biological difference between papillary and nodular carcinomas by polymerase chain reaction (PCR)/single-strand conformation of polymorphism (SSCP) analysis (Fujimoto et al in press). This method is efficient in detecting base changes in determined sequences of DNA (Saiki et al 1985, Orita et al 1989) and we examined whether or not tumour progression is characterized by p53 gene alteration in human bladder cancers. Twenty-three specimens of bladder cancer, 22 TCC and 1 squamous cell

Table 3.1 p53 gene mutation in human bladder cancer

	Bladder cancer specimens	Histopathological stage	grade[a]	p53 gene mutation exon	codon	amino acid change
Superficial carcinoma	3T	pTaN0M0	G_2		n.d.[b]	
	4T	pTaN0m0	G_2		n.d.	
	6T	pTaN0M0	G_2		n.d.	
	9T	pT1N0M0	G_2		n.d.	
	10T	pT1N0M0	G_3		n.d.	
	11Tis	pTis[c] in pT3bN4M0	G_3	exon 8	270	Phe(TTT) → Val(GTT)
	13T	pTaN0M0	G_1		n.d.	
	14T	pT1N0M0	G_3		n.d.	
	15T	pTaN0M0	G_2		n.d.	
	16T	pTaN0M0	G_1		n.d.	
	17T	pT1N0M0	G_2		n.d.	
	21T	pT1N0M0	G_3		n.d.	
	23T	pTaN0M0	G_1		n.d.	
Invasive carcinoma	1T	pT3N0M0	G_2		n.d.	
	2T	pT3bN0M0	G_3		n.d.	
	5T	pT3bN1M0	G_3		n.d.	
	7T	pT3N0M0	G_3	exon 5	159	Ala(GCC) → Pro(CCC)
	8T	pT2N0M0	G_3	exon 8	280	Frameshift caused by 1bp insertion Arg(AGA) → Thr(ACG)
	11T	pT3bN4M0	G_3		n.d.	
	11M	pT3bN4M0	G_3	exon 8	270	Phe(TTT) → Val(GTT)
	12T[d]	pT3bN0M0	G_3	exon 4	104–110 or –111	21bp deletion
	18T	pT4N4M0	G_3	exon 4	43	Leu(TTG) → Ser(TCG)
	19T	pT3N0M0	G_3		n.d.	
	20T	pT3bN1M0	G_3	exon 5	158	Arg(CGC) → His(CAC)
	22T	pT3N1M1	G_3	exon 9	327 or 328	Stop codon at codon 344 caused by 1bp deletion

(*a*) classified under the provision of the General Rule for Clinical and Pathological Studies on Bladder Cancer (Japanese Urological Association and the Japanese Pathological Society 1980) (*b*) not detected (*c*) carcinoma in situ (flat tumour) (*d*) this specimen consisted of squamous cell carcinoma alone without any transitional cell carcinoma component anywhere in the urinary bladder and other organs. Reproduced with permission from Fujimoto et al 1992 (in press).

carcinoma, were obtained at either cystectomy or TUR, frozen in liquid nitrogen, and stored at −80°C. DNA was extracted from tissue by proteinase K digestion and phenol/chloroform extraction.

As primers for PCR, oligonucleotides were synthesized on the basis of the published p53 gene sequences in each region from exon 4 to 11. One hundred ng of genomic DNA was amplified in a total volume of 25 μl buffer and 0.1 U Taq polymerase. Thirty cycles of reaction at 94, 55, and 72°C for 30, 30 and 60 seconds, respectively, were run in a DNA Thermal Cycler. Two μl of PCR product was diluted 100–fold with a buffer and heated at 80°C for two minutes. One μl of this solution was then applied to a 6% neutral polyacrylamide gel on each lane. Electrophoresis was performed at 30 W for 1 to 6 hours, depending on the length of an amplified nucleotide. The gel was dried and exposed to X-ray film at −80°C for 2–24 hours with an intensifying screen. Of 13 superficial bladder cancers (pTis, pTa and pT1), none had p53 gene mutation except for one CIS, whereas 6 of 10 nodular invasive cancers (pT2 and pT3) had p53 gene mutations, as shown in Table 3.1.

CONCLUSION

Cancer arises by the accumulation of genetic alterations, and the multi-step process has been elucidated, for example, in colon carcinogenesis (Vogelstein et al 1988, Nishisho et al 1991) and, as reviewed here, bladder carcinogenesis. Such molecular information is very important in considering clinicobiological features of bladder cancer, inhibition of bladder carcinogenesis at an appropriate step in relation to tumour recurrences and progression, prediction of malignant progression, and the development of new molecular markers for both monitoring and early detection. Further detailed molecular information relating to bladder cancer is required.

REFERENCES

Abel P D, Hall P R, Williams G 1988 Should pT1 transitional cell cancers of the bladder still be classified as superficial? Br J Urol 62: 235–239

Birch B R P, Harland, S J 1989 Review: The pT1 G3 bladder tumor. Br J Urol 64: 109–116

Droller M J 1986 Transitional cell cancer: upper tracts and bladder. In: Walsh P C, Gittes R F, Perlmutter A D et al (eds) Campbell's urology. Saunders, Philadelphia. p 1343

Fearon E R, Feinberg A P, Hamilton S H et al 1985 Loss of genes on the short arm of chromosome 11 in bladder cancer. Nature 318: 377–380

Feinberg A P, Vogelstein B, Droller M J et al 1983 Mutation affecting the 12th amino acid of the c-Ha-ras oncogene product occurs infrequently in human cancer. Science 220: 1175–1177

Friedell G H, Soloway M S, Hilgar A G et al 1986 Summary of workshop on carcinoma in situ of the bladder. J Urol 136: 1047–1048

Fujimoto K, Yamada Y, Okajima E et al 1992 Frequent association of p53 gene mutation in invasive bladder cancer. Cancer Res, in press

Fujita J, Srivastava S K, Kraus M H et al 1985 Frequency of molecular alterations affecting ras protooncogenes in human urinary tract tumors. Proc Natl Acad Sci USA 82: 3849–3853

Green L F, Hanash K A, Farrow G M 1973 Benign papilloma or papillary carcinoma of the bladder? J Urol 110: 205–207
Heney N M, Ahmed S, Flanagan M et al 1983 Superficial bladder cancer: progression and recurrence. J Urol 130: 1083–1086
Jakse G, Loidl W, Seeber G et al 1987 Stage T1, grade 3 transitional cell carcinoma of the bladder: an unfavorable tumor? J Urol 137: 39–43
Kakizoe T, Matsumoto K, Nishio Y et al 1984 Analysis of 90 step-sectioned cystectomized specimens of bladder cancer. J Urol 131: 467–472
Kakizoe T, Tobisu K, Takai K et al 1988 Relationship between papillary and nodular transitional cell carcinoma in the human urinary bladder. Cancer Res 48: 2293–2303
Lamb D 1967 Correlation of chromosome counts with histological appearances and prognosis in transitional-cell carcinoma of the bladder. BMJ 1: 273–377
Lerner S P, Tsai Y C, Jones P A 1991 Genetic aspects of bladder cancer progression. World Journal of Urology 9: 69–74
Lam B L, Torti F M 1991 Adjuvant intravesicular pharmacotherapy for superficial bladder cancer. J Nat Cancer Inst 83: 682–694
Milasin J, Micic M, Micic S et al 1987 Ring chromosomes in bladder cancer. Cancer Genet Cytogenet 28: 183–184
Murphy V M, Emerson L D, Chandler R W et al 1986 Flow cytometry versus urinary cytology in the evaluation of patients with bladder cancer. J Urol 136: 815–819
Nishisho I, Nakamura Y, Miyoshi Y et al 1991 Mutations of chromosome 5q21 genes in FAP and colorectal cancer patients. Science 253: 665–669
Olumi A F, Tsai Y C, Nicholas P W et al 1990 Allelic loss of chromosome 17p distinguishes high grade from low grade transitional cell carcinomas of the bladder. Cancer Res 50: 7081–7083
Orita M, Iwahana H, Kanazawa H et al 1989 Detection of polymorphisms of human DNA by gel electrophoresis as single-strand conformation polymorphisms. Proc Natl Acad Sci USA 86: 2766–2770
Pagano F, Garbeglio A, Milani C et al 1987 Prognosis of bladder cancer. Eur Urol 13: 145–149
Reddy E P, Reynolds R K, Santos E et al 1982 A point mutation is responsible for the acquisition of transforming properties by the T24 human bladder carcinoma oncogene. Nature 300: 149–152
Saiki R K, Scharf S, Faloona S et al 1985 Enzymatic amplification of β-globin genomic sequences and restriction site analysis for diagnosis of sickle cell anemia. Science 230: 1350–1354
Sandberg A A 1977 Chromosome markers and progression in bladder cancer. Cancer Res 37: 2950–2956
Sidransky D, Eschenbach A V, Tsai Y C et al 1991 Identification of p53 gene mutations in bladder cancers and urine samples. Science 252: 706–709
Spooner M E, Cooper E H 1972 Chromosome constitution of transitional cell carcinoma of the urinary bladder. Cancer 29: 1401–1412
Summers J L, Falor W H, Ward R 1981 A 10–year analysis of chromosomes in noninvasive papillary carcinoma of the bladder. J Urol 125: 177–178
Tabin C J, Bradley S M, Bargmann C I et al 1982 Mechanism of activation of a human oncogene. Nature 300: 143–149
Tsai Y C, Nichols P W, Hiti A L et al 1990 Allelic losses of chromosomes 9, 11, and 17 in human bladder cancer. Cancer Res 50: 44–47
Vogelstein B, Fearon E R, Hamilton S R et al 1988 Genetic alterations during colorectal tumor development. N Engl J Med 319: 525–532

4. Genetic steps associated with prostate cancer development

M. J. G. Bussemakers F. M. J. Debruyne
J. A. Schalken

INTRODUCTION

Prostate cancer is an increasing medical problem: it is now the most commonly diagnosed cancer in the Western male population and the second leading cause of cancer deaths in man (Boring et al 1991). Despite the increasing number of patients that manifest with clinical disease, little is known about the mechanisms involved in the onset and progression of prostate cancer. However, it seems clear that prostate carcinogenesis is a multistep process leading first to histological prostate cancers that upon acquisition of additional malignant events develop into clinical disease (Carter et al 1990). During the change of tumour phenotype from benign to malignant and eventually metastatic state, an accumulation of genetic changes (qualitative as well as quantitative) occurs (Nicolson 1991). This often provides the target cell with the ability to circumvent controls that regulate growth, thereby gaining the propensity to proliferate indefinitely. This increased proliferative capacity has two important consequences. First, there is an increased chance of the acquisition of genetic hits due to the fact that most genotoxic agents damage genes in cycling cells. Second, this increased proliferative capacity is required for the outgrowth of the malignant population of cells. Genes implicated in uncontrolled proliferation are often identified as oncogenes or tumour suppressor genes. Progression to the more malignant state, i.e. acquisition of metastatic ability, requires that the cell can invade the surrounding tissue, spread through the lymphatic and/or blood circulation, extravasate and grow at secondary sites, a process usually involving changes in other genes such as those implicated in proteolysis, cell adhesion and cell motility.

The identification of the genetic steps associated with the onset and progression of cancer is now a focus of molecular oncological research. The tremendous developments in molecular biology and immunology in recent years have provided a wide variety of tools to identify and study the target genes implicated in prostate carcinogenesis. Whereas a genetic cascade for the development of colon cancer development is now emerging (Fearon & Vogelstein 1990), the situation for prostate cancer is still unclear. Moreover, morphological changes occurring in the aetiology of prostate cancer

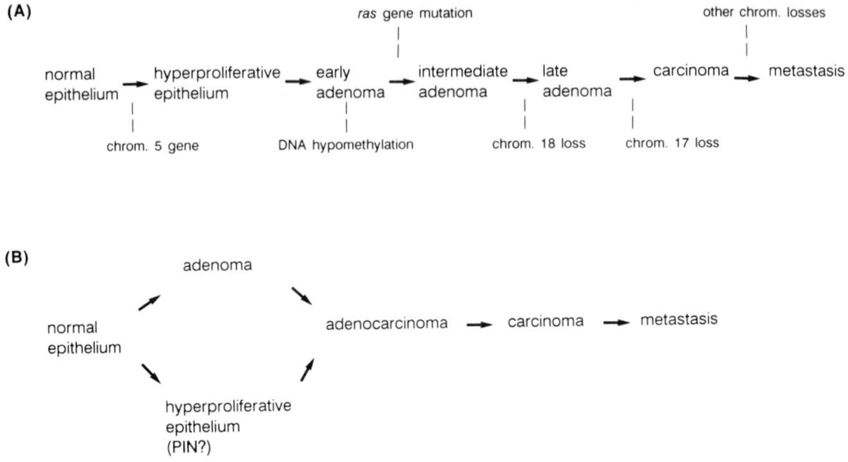

Fig. 4.1 **A** Molecular steps associated with the progression of colorectal cancer. **B** Progressional stages in prostate cancer. The genetic events associated with these stages remain to be established.

are not unequivocally recognized, i.e. can we identify a hyperproliferative stage in development that precedes the outgrowth into an adenocarcinoma, a carcinoma and a metastatic tumour? (Fig. 4.1). The occurrence of specific genetic changes and their place (i.e. early versus late event) in this cascade is not yet understood. This chapter reviews the results to date regarding the molecular steps associated with prostate cancer. We discuss first the 'indirect approach', the study of known genes with potential relevance for cancer development, and then the 'direct approach' aimed at the characterization of molecular differences between aggressive and non-aggressive cancers. Finally, we will discuss the potential of molecular biology in advanced diagnostics.

THE 'INDIRECT APPROACH': STUDY OF KNOWN GENES WITH POTENTIAL RELEVANCE FOR CANCER DEVELOPMENT

GENES IMPLICATED IN CELL GROWTH

The most striking advantage a cancer cell has over a non-cancer cell is its unlimited growth potential which is presumably associated with a corrupted cell cycle control. Basic studies on the mechanisms of growth control might give us clues as to which genes are implicated in the onset and progression of cancer. Several groups of genes are involved in growth control. To gain insight into which of these genes are implicated in carcinogenesis, one has to consider several hundreds of genes such as (proto)-oncogenes, tumour suppressor genes, and genes encoding growth factors, growth factor receptors, and transcription factors.

Oncogenes and tumour suppressor genes

For prostate cancer several proto-oncogenes have been studied at different levels: proto-oncogenes can be activated to oncogenes by mutations (qualitative changes) but also by changes in mRNA or protein expression levels (quantitative changes) (Nicolson 1991). The possible involvement of the ras-family of oncogenes and proteins were extensively studied for prostate cancer. Peehl and associates (1987) reported on the presence of an activated Ki-ras oncogene in a primary prostate cancer. Recently, however, it was shown that the frequency of ras-mutations in prostate cancer is rather low (Carter et al 1990a, Gumerlock et al 1991). Studies at the ras mRNA level in the Dunning rat prostate adenocarcinoma model system showed no clear correlation of overexpression of the ras-oncogenes with tumour progression (Cooke et al 1988b, Bussemakers et al 1991a), nor did studies in human prostatic carcinoma cell lines (Rijnders et al 1985). Viola et al (1986) studied the ras gene product, p21, and showed an inverse relation between $p21^{ras}$ and histological tumour grade. Furthermore, $p21^{ras}$ levels correlated with the frequency of nodal metastases. However, the monoclonal antibody used in these experiments was shown to be nonspecific in subsequent studies (Samowitz et al 1988). More recently, Sumiya et al (1990) found a higher expression of $p21^{ras}$ in high-grade and high-stage tumours, although in high-stage tumours $p21^{ras}$ expression did not correlate with survival. Several other oncogenes were studied at the mRNA level in the Dunning model system (Cooke et al 1988a, Bussemakers et al 1991a) and in human prostatic carcinoma cell lines (Rijnders et al 1985) but no clear correlation of expression of any of the oncogenes studied with tumour progression was shown. Interestingly, Fleming et al (1986) and Buttyan et al (1987) found increased levels of myc expression in high-grade prostate cancers. The implications of these findings are still unclear.

Until now, no consistent genetic changes affecting (proto-)oncogenes are evident for prostate cancer. Similarly, no consistent genetic changes are found in tumour suppressor genes. Point mutations in p53, a tumour suppressor gene shown to be involved in several human cancers, were shown to be rare in human prostate cancers, although in several prostate cell lines mutations in p53 were found (Isaacs et al 1991). Loss of retinoblastoma (Rb) gene expression, presumably associated with a promoter deletion, was found in only one out of seven human prostate cancers, and in one out of three cell lines, suggesting that Rb mutations are not common in prostate cancer. However, reintroduction of a normal Rb gene into DU145 cells (human prostate cancer cell line with a mutated Rb gene) resulted in the reversion of the tumorigenic phenotype of the cells (Bookstein et al 1990).

In conclusion, ras and p53 mutations are far less frequently found in prostate cancer than in other solid tumours. However, future studies have to reveal whether prostate tumours containing ras and/or p53 mutations represent more aggressive subpopulations.

Growth factors and growth factor receptors

The prostate is known to contain large amounts of growth factors such as basic fibroblast growth factor (bFGF), transforming growth factor-β (TGF-β), transforming growth factor-α (TGF-α) and epidermal growth factor (EGF). Also, the receptors for these growth factors are present in the prostate gland (reviewed by Thompson 1990). Studies by Mori and associates (1990) showed that bFGF is expressed at elevated levels in benign prostate hyperplasia (BPH) as compared to normal prostatic tissue, suggesting that this growth factor might be involved in benign growth disorders of the human prostate. The fact that bFGF has been shown to be mitogenic to cultured prostate epithelial cells (McKeehan et al 1987) provides additional evidence for a possible role of bFGF in abnormal growth of the prostate. TGF-β2 is also expressed at elevated levels in BPH as compared to normal prostate (Mori et al 1990). TGF-β1 is highly expressed in poorly-differentiated rat prostate tumours when compared to well-differentiated tumours (Wilding et al 1989). Considering its ability to induce angiogenesis (Roberts et al 1986), cell motility (Myrdal et al 1986) and deposition of the extracellular matrix (Rizzino 1988), TGF-β1 might contribute to a more malignant phenotype (see below). EGF is expressed in both normal and malignant prostate tissue, but the elevated levels of EGF-receptor and mRNA (Morris & Dodd 1990) in human prostate cancers when compared to normal prostate, might indicate a role for EGF in the complex process of prostate carcinogenesis.

A unique feature of the prostate gland is its dependence on androgens. Furthermore, growth and differentiation of benign and malignant prostatic epithelial cells are regulated by androgens. This suggests an important role for androgens and the androgen receptor in prostate carcinogenesis. Experiments have shown the androgen-regulated DNA synthesis in the ventral prostate (Coffey & Williams-Ashman 1968), and some genes encoding growth factors and some non-growth-factor proto-oncogenes are under androgenic control. Androgen ablation (by castration) leading to an active process of cell death, is associated with increased levels of c-myc, c-fos and TGFβ1 mRNA (Buttyan et al 1988, Kyprianou & Isaacs 1989) and also an increased number of receptor binding sites for TGFβ1 and EGF (Kyprianou & Isaacs 1988, St. Arnaud et al 1988). Upon castration and readministration of androgens, transient increases in steady-state levels of several genes like c-Ha-ras, c-Ki-ras, c-myc, c-fos and bFGF have been observed (Katz et al 1989). These results suggest a complex regulation of gene expression by androgens and indicate that inappropriate androgenic regulation of proto-oncogenes and growth factors may contribute to the progression of prostate cancer. A role for the androgen receptor in prostate cancer has not been established: using monoclonal antibodies it was shown that loss of androgen receptor expression is not associated with the progression of prostate cancer. No correlation with tumour grade or stage was evident (Van der Kwast et al 1991).

The importance of a diffusable factor or factors synthesized in response to androgens by prostate stromal cells was already reported by Cunha et al (1983). Tissue recombination studies indicated that these factors induce the proliferation and/or differentiation of prostate epithelial cells. Using this technique, Chung and associates (1989) showed that fibroblasts can play a role in the development of prostate cancer. They also showed that the expression of six extracellular matrix genes was decreased upon transformation (Freeman et al 1991), suggesting the involvement not only of paracrine growth factors but also of the extracellular matrix in prostate carcinogenesis (see below). Additional evidence for the presence of diffusible factors was reported by Djakiew and colleagues (1990), who showed the stimulation of prostate epithelial cell growth by factors secreted by prostate stromal cells. Furthermore, paracrine growth stimulation is implicated not only in local growth of the prostate but also in the formation of metastases: PC3 cells were shown to secrete a factor that stimulates the growth of bone cells, indicating that this factor might play a role in osteoblastic metastases as seen in prostatic cancer (Perkel et al 1990).

GENES IMPLICATED IN INVASION AND METASTASIS

During the progression of a tumour to a metastatic state, cancer cells have to acquire the ability to invade locally into small blood vessels and/or lymphatic systems. If the cells survive the host defence/surveillance mechanisms, they have to extravasate and move into surrounding organ tissue and finally proliferate to give rise to clinical apparent metastases (Hart et al 1989). The acquisition of metastatic properties is probably due to changes in the expression of genes involved in cell attachment and cell motility. One might expect increasing levels of degradative enzymes (such as proteases) or decreasing levels of their inhibitors (such as tissue inhibitors of metalloproteinases; TIMP); The expression levels of cell adhesion molecules may change, and the expression of components that aid the cells in escaping host defence mechanisms may also be important. For prostate cancer, the genes involved in the acquisition of metastatic ability are largely unknown. Of the genes that might be important in cell attachment and cell motility, only a few were studied: increased levels of plasminogen activors were shown in human prostatic cancers (Gaylis et al 1989) and in rat model systems (Wilson et al 1990); secretion of collagenase by a rat prostatic epidermoid carcinoma in culture has been reported (Huang et al 1979); and elevated activities of elastase and a chymotrypsin-like protease were found in metastatic Dunning tumours (Lowe & Isaacs 1984). Recently, it was shown that E-cadherin, a calcium-dependent cell adhesion molecule, is down-regulated in invasive prostate cancers (Bussemakers et al 1991c). The association of changes in the expression of different components of the extracellular matrix with a transformed phenotype of rat prostate fibroblasts (Freeman et al 1991) has already been mentioned. For completeness, it should be mentioned that fibronectin is down-modulated in metastatic prostate cancer cells (Schalken et al 1988), although these results were obtained by a direct approach (differential hybridization analysis).

THE 'DIRECT APPROACH': IDENTIFICATION OF MOLECULAR CHARACTERISTICS OF PROGRESSIONALLY ADVANCED PROSTATE CANCER CELLS

LOSS OF HETEROZYGOSITY

The low mitotic index of prostate tumours and the difficulty in growing prostate cancers in culture, has made studies of chromosomal changes associated with the onset and progression of prostate cancer rather difficult. Nonetheless, the involvement of some specific chromosomal changes have thus been identified. As summarized by Brothman and associates (1990), loss of chromosomes 1, 2, 5, 11 and Y, trisomy of chromosomes 7, 14, 20 and 22, and structural changes involving chromosomal segments 2p, 7q and 10q are the most common changes reported. Of these, deletions of 7q and 10q were found in late-stage cancers (Atkin & Baker 1985a,b). However, all these findings are based on small numbers of patients. A less complicated technique that overcomes the problems associated with the low mitotic index in prostate cancer, is allelotyping. Using DNA probes that recognize restriction fragment length polymorphisms (RFLPs), one can identify deletions of (parts of) chromosomes. Using this technique, the frequent deletion of the long arm of chromosome 17 in colon cancer was revealed, leading to the identification of p53 as a potential tumour suppressor gene (Baker et al 1989). Also, a candidate tumour suppressor gene on chromosome 18 was identified after an initial lead obtained from RFLP analysis (Fearon et al 1990). RFLP analysis now provides a technique to test the observations on chromosome deletion in prostate cancer mentioned above in a large group of patients and also to include all known chromosomal loci thus far reported to contain potential tumour suppressor genes. Carter et al (1990b) showed that whereas the loss of chromosome 10 did indeed frequently occur (30% of cases studied), an as yet unreported loss of chromosome 16 was observed more frequently. These results suggest that chromosomes 10q and 16q should be studied in more detail to identify a relation between allelic loss and progression of the tumour and to identify candidate tumour suppressor genes located on these chromosomes.

MONOCLONAL ANTIBODIES

The development of hybridoma technology (Kohler & Milstein 1975) offered the ability to produce antibodies detecting specific antigens. Using tumour cell extracts, and upon appropriate screening, it is possible to raise antibodies against tumour-specific antigens. Although the use of monoclonal antibodies as progression markers is established in many disciplines, for prostate cancer it is still an underexplored approach. While the isolation of several prostate cancer monoclonal antibodies was reported (Webb et al 1984, Lindgren et al 1985, Starling et al 1986), none were shown to be useful as progression markers. Although TURP–27 (Starling et al 1986) has only limited value as a progression marker, it was interesting to learn that the antigens recognized by this antibody are related to those recognized by HNK–1 (Lipford & Wright 1991). HNK–1 recognizes antigens related to the neural cell adhesion molecule (N-CAM). Recently, a new monoclonal antibody specific to prostate cancer, PD41 has been described (Beckett et al 1991). Its value for diagnosis and the nature of the antigen remain to be established.

DIFFERENTIAL HYBRIDIZATION ANALYSIS

Another direct approach to identify molecular differences associated with prostate tumour development is based on the comparison of steady-state mRNA populations. These techniques, such as differential or subtraction hybridization, enable the identification of genes expressed at different levels but do not allow the identification of genes aberrantly expressed. Differential or subtraction hybridization analysis have several advantages: one can screen for genes which are up-regulated as well as down-regulated; the reagents which become available, i.e. cDNA clones, are easy to characterize by DNA sequence analysis and computer-assisted database comparison; finally, usefulness of the reagent in diagnosis can be evaluated immediately by RNA in-situ hybridization. These techniques have been successfully used in identifying genes induced by growth factors (Lau & Nathans 1985, 1987; Almendral et al 1988) or genes differentially expressed when comparing normal versus malignant tissue (Augentlich et al 1982, Matrisian et al 1986). For metastasis, few reports are available, most of them reporting on down-regulation of gene expression during progression. In melanoma cells with low metastatic potential, NM23 is down-regulated (Steeg et al 1988); in metastatic mammary adenocarcinoma WDNM1 and -2 are down-regulated (Dear et al 1988, 1989); and for rat metastasizing prostate cancer cells a down-modulation of fibronectin was shown (Schalken et al 1988). These results indicate that, as in tumorigenesis, suppressor genes might also be involved in metastasis (metastasis suppressor genes). For prostate cancer, we recently identified two cDNA clones that are overexpressed in metastatic rat prostate cancers (Bussemakers et al 1991b). One of these was found to be rather specific for metastasizing tumours, and upon DNA sequence analysis was shown to be identical or related to high mobility group protein I (Y) (HMG-I(Y)). This protein is a small, non-histone nuclear protein implicated in transcription and replication processes. Its overexpression in dedifferentiated, fast-proliferating cells was reported earlier (Johnson et al 1988). The value of HMG-I(Y) as a progression marker needs further investigation. The second cDNA clone contained rat-specific LTR-like sequences and is not likely to be useful for human diagnosis. Interestingly, Liu & Abraham (1991), studying differential gene expression in human prostatic cancer cell lines, identified a cDNA containing human endogenous retroviral sequences spliced to human calbindin. The possible role of retroviral sequences in prostate cancer, however, remains unclear.

DISCUSSION AND PERSPECTIVES

The major questions in prostate cancer, i.e. what is the cellular origin of cancer and which molecular steps are implicated in its development, are still essentially open. There are some indications of the importance of as yet unidentified tumour suppressor genes, and several progression markers are under investigation. However, the question remains as to whether these markers can be used in a routine setting or whether they will require more advanced technology.

INTERPHASE CYTOGENETICS

The frequent loss of chromosomes 10 and 16 might prove to be useful progression markers in prostate cancer diagnosis. Since RFLP analysis is a technique with little feasibility in a pathological setting, interphase cytogenetics might be a better approach (Hopman et al 1988). This technique involves the in-situ hybridization of interphase nuclei using chromosome-specific probes, and enables the study of numerical chromosomal aberrations. Thus, a study on a large group of patients with superficial bladder cancer showed the frequent loss of chromosome 9 and the frequent gain of chromosome 1 (Hopman et al 1991). Until now, the chromosome-specific probes used often recognized the centromeric region of the chromosome, thereby preventing the detection of arm deletions. The use of cosmid clones might enable the analysis of more specific regions for over/under representation of the genome in cancer cells. Of further importance for interphase cytogenetics is the definition of the area of interest, especially considering the tumour cell heterogeneity in prostate cancer. Since it is not yet clear whether reliable in-situ interphase cytogenetics (i.e. on frozen- and paraffin-embedded sections) will be possible, the nuclei preparations need to be made from pathologically defined sections. However, the technique is potentially powerful in the study of gross genetic aberrations associated with prostate tumour progression.

RNA IN-SITU HYBRIDIZATION

Progression markers identified by differential/subtraction hybridization analysis, are isolated as cDNA clones. If they represent known genes, and if antibodies against these genes are available, immunohistochemical studies can be performed – on fresh and/or archival material – to establish the importance of these progression markers. If, however, an unknown gene is identified or if an antibody is not available, one might consider RNA in-situ hybridization to study primary prostate samples. Since RNA molecules are extremely sensitive to degradation, the use of RNA in-situ hybridization requires careful tissue handling. This aspect of the technique may impair its use in a routine setting.

POLYMERASE CHAIN REACTION

The polymerase chain reaction (PCR) technique has many applications and many publications have already shown its potential (see Ehrlich 1989 for a review). The technique is based on the exponential amplification of small amounts of target sequences, and one needs only a small amount of material in contrast to most standard protocols. For a diagnostic approach one might even consider the use of tissue-sections (Coates et al 1991). PCR is a largely simple procedure; however an adequate choice of primers is of great importance and, since the technique is very sensitive, minor contaminations may interfere with the results of the experiment. Also, quantification of the amplification is still cumbersome.

Recently, two methods have been developed, enabling the (relatively easy) detection of point mutations. Single strand conformation polymorphism PCR (SSCP-PCR) is based on the fact that single-stranded DNA when run under non-denaturing conditions forms a secondary conformation that will change due to (point) mutations (Orita et al 1989). The various conformations have a different motility in a non-denaturing gel and can be discriminated accordingly. Thus, Suzuki et al (1990) studied a great number of mutations in the *ras*-oncogene. When studying a gene with known hot-spots for mutation, the technique can be extremely useful to analyse large numbers of patients. The second technique, denaturing gradient gel electrophoresis (DGGE), is based on the fact that, due to changes in nucleotide sequence, DNA-fragments have different melting point characteristics which can be visualized when run in a denaturing gel (Meyers et al 1987). Recently, the slightly modified technique of constant denaturant gel electrophoresis (CDGE), was used to rapidly screen for p53 mutations in breast carcinomas (Børresen et al 1991). Considering the many applications and possibilities of the technique, PCR-based technology is likely to become a routine instrument in molecular (uro)pathological analysis.

In conclusion, there are at present only a few markers available with potential use in the prediction of the metastatic ability of prostate cancer cells. Considering the increasing number of patients diagnosed with prostate cancer, the identification of additional molecular markers for prostate cancer is of great importance. Also, the development and/or improvement of discriminative screening techniques that can be used in a routine setting is required; i.e. future studies should aim at a screening program for prostate cancer which makes possible prediction of the aggressiveness of the individual tumour.

REFERENCES

Almendral J M, Sommer D, Macdonald-Bravo H et al 1988 Complexity of the early genetic response to growth factors in mouse fibroblasts. Mol Cell Biol 8: 2140–2148

Atkin N B, Baker M C 1985a Chromosome 10 deletion in carcinoma of the prostate. N Engl J Med 312: 315

Atkin N B, Baker M C 1985b Chromosome study of five cancers of the prostate. Hum Genet 70: 359–364

Augentlicht L H, Kobrin D 1982 Cloning and screening of sequences expressed in a mouse colon tumor. Cancer Res 42: 1088–1093

Baker S J, Fearon E R, Nigro J M et al 1989 Chromosomes 17 deletions and p53 mutations in colorectal carcinomas. Science 244: 217–221

Beckett M L, Lipford G B, Haley C L et al 1991 Monoclonal antibody PD41 recognizes an antigen restricted to prostate adenocarcinomas. Cancer Res 51: 1326–1333

Bookstein R, Shew J-Y, Chen P-L et al 1990 Suppression of tumorigenicity of human prostate carcinoma cells by replacing a mutated RB gene. Science 247: 712–715

Boring C C, Squires T S, Tong T 1991 Cancer Statistics, 1991. CA Cancer J Clin 41: 19–36

Børresen A-L, Hovig E, Smith-Sørensen B et al 1991 Constant denaturant gel electrophoresis as a rapid screening technique for p53 mutations. Proc Natl Acad Sci USA 88: 8405–8409

Brothman A R, Peehl D M, Patel A M et al 1990 Frequency and pattern of karyotypic abnormalities in human prostate cancer. Cancer Res 50: 3795–3803

Bussemakers M J G, Isaacs J T, Debruyne F M J et al 1991a Oncogene expression in prostate cancer. World Journal of Urology 9: 58–63

Bussemakers M J G, Van de Ven W J M, Debruyne F M J et al 1991b Identification of high mobility group protein I (Y) as a potential marker for prostate cancer by differential hybridization analysis. Cancer Res 51: 606–611

Bussemakers M J G, Van Moorselaar R J A, Giroldi L A et al 1991c Decreased expression of E-cadherin in rat prostate cancer cells. Submitted

Buttyan R, Sawczuk I S, Benson M C et al 1987 Enhanced expression of the c-*myc* protooncogene in high-grade human prostate cancers. Prostate 11: 327–337

Buttyan R, Zakeri Z, Lockshin R et al 1988 Cascade induction of c-*fos*, c-*myc*, and heat-shock 70 K transcripts during regression of the rat ventral prostate. Mol Endocrinol 2: 650–657

Carter B S, Epstein J I, Isaacs W B 1990a *Ras* gene mutations in human prostate cancer. Cancer Res 50: 6830–6832

Carter B S, Ewing C M, Ward W S et al 1990b Allelic loss of chromosomes 16q and 10q in human prostate cancer. Proc Natl Acad Sci USA 87: 8751–8755

Carter H B, Piantadosi S, Isaacs J T 1990 Clinical evidence for and implications of the multistep development of prostate cancer. J Urol 143: 742–746

Chung L W K, Chang S-M, Bell C et al 1989 Co-inoculation of tumorigenic rat prostate mesenchymal cells with non-tumorigenic epithelial cells results in the development of carcinosarcoma in syngeneic and athymic animals. Int J Cancer 43: 1179–1187

Coates P J, D'Ardenne A J, Khan G et al 1991 Simplified procedures for applying the polymerase chain reaction to routinely fixed paraffin wax sections. J Clin Pathol 44: 115–118

Coffey D S, Williams-Ashman H G 1968 Polymerization of deoxyribonucleotides in relation to androgen-induced prostate growth. Arch Biochem Biophys 124: 184–198

Cooke D B, Quarmby V E, Mickey D D et al 1988a Oncogene expression in prostate cancer: Dunning R-3327 rat dorsal prostatic adenocarcinoma system. Prostate 13: 263–272

Cooke D B, Quarmby V E, Petrusz P 1988b Expression of *ras* proto-oncogenes in the Dunning R-3327 rat prostatic adenocarcinoma system. Prostate 13: 273–288

Cunha G R, Chung L W K, Shannon J M et al 1983 Hormone-induced morphogenesis and growth: role of mesenchymal-epithelial interactions. Recent Prog Horm Res 39: 559–598

Dear T N, Ramshaw I A, Kefford R F 1988 Differential expression of a novel gene, WDNM1, in nonmetastatic rat mammary adenomarcinoma cells. Cancer Res 48: 5203–5209

Dear T N, McDonald D A, Kefford R F 1989 Transcriptional down-regulation of a rat gene, WDNM2, in metastatic DMBA-8 cells. Cancer Res 49: 5323–5328

Djakiew D, Tarkington M A, Lynch J H 1990 Paracrine stimulation of polarized secretion from monolayers of a neoplastic prostatic epithelial cell line by prostatic stromal cell proteins. Cancer Res 50: 1966–1974

Ehrlich H A 1989 PCR technology: principles and applications for DNA amplification. Stockton Press, New York

Fearon E R, Vogelstein B 1990 A genetic model for colorectal tumorigenesis. Cell 61: 759–767

Fearon E R, Cho K R, Nigro J M et al 1990 Identification of a chromosome 18q gene that is altered in colorectal carcinomas. Science 247: 49–56

Fleming W H, Hamel A, MacDonald R et al 1986 Expression of the c-*myc* protooncogene in human prostatic carcinoma and benign prostatic hyperplasia. Cancer Res 46: 1535–1538

Freeman M R, Song Y, Carson D D et al 1991 Extracellular matrix and androgen receptor expression associated with spontaneous transformation of rat prostate fibroblasts. Cancer Res 51: 1910–1916

Gaylis F D, Keer H N, Wilson M J et al 1989 Plasminogen activators in human prostate cancer cell lines and tumors: correlation with the aggressive phenotype. J Urol 142: 193–198

Gumerlock P H, Poonamallee U R, Meyers F J et al 1991 Activated *ras* alleles in human carcinoma of the prostate are rare. Cancer Res 51: 1632–1637

Hart I R, Goode N T, Wilson R E 1989 Molecular aspects of the metastatic cascade. Biochim Biophys Acta 989: 65–84

Hopman A H N, Ramaekers F C S, Raap A K et al 1988 in situ hybridization as a tool to study numerical chromosomal aberrations in solid bladder tumors. Histochemistry 89: 307–316

Hopman A H N, Moesker O, Smeets A W C B et al 1991 Numerical chromosome 1, 7, 9 and 11 aberrations in bladder cancer detected by in situ hybridization. Cancer Res 51: 644–651

Huang C-C, Wu C-H, Abramson M 1979 Collagenase activity in cultures of rat prostate carcinoma. Biochim Biophys Acta 570: 149–156

Isaacs W B, Carter B S, Ewing C M 1991 Wild type p53 suppresses growth of human cancer cells containing mutant p53 alleles. Cancer Res 51: 4716–4720

Johnson K R, Lehn D A, Elton T S et al 1988 Complete murine cDNA sequence, genomic structure, and tissue expression of the high mobility group protein HMG-I(Y). J Biol Chem 263: 18338–18342

Katz A E, Benson M C, Wise G J et al 1989 Gene activity during the early phase of androgen-stimulated rat prostate regrowth. Cancer Res 49: 5889–5894

Kohler G, Milstein G 1975 Continuous cultures of fused cells secreting antibody of predefined specificity. Nature 265: 493–495

Kyprianou N, Isaacs J T 1988 Identification of a cellular receptor for transforming growth factor-β in rat ventral prostate and its negative regulation by androgens. Endocrinology 123: 2124–2131

Kyprianou N, Isaacs J T 1989 Expression of transforming growth factor-β in the rat ventral prostate during castration-induced programmed cell death. Mol Endocrinol 3: 1515–1522

Lau L F, Nathans D 1985 Identification of a set of genes expressed during G0/G1 transition of cultured mouse cells. EMBO J 4: 3145–3151

Lau L F, Nathans D 1987 Expression of a set of growth-related immediate early genes in Balb/c 3T3 cells: coordinate regulation with c-*fos* or c-*myc*. Proc Natl Acad Sci USA 84: 1182–1186

Lindgren J, Pak K Y, Ernst C et al 1985 Shared antigens of human prostate cancer cell lines as defined by monoclonal antibodies. Hybridoma 4: 37–45

Lipford G B, Wright Jr G L 1991 Comparative study of monoclonal antibodies TURP–27 and HNK–1: their relationship to neural cell adhesion molecules and prostate tumor-associated antigens. Cancer Res 51: 2296–2301

Liu A Y, Abrahan B A 1991 Subtractive cloning of a hybrid human endogenous retrovirus and calbindin gene in the prostate cell line PC3. Cancer Res 51: 4107–4110

Lowe F C, Isaacs J T 1984 Biochemical methods for predicting metastatic ability of prostatic cancer utilizing the Dunning R–3327 rat prostatic adenocarcinoma system as a model. Cancer Res 44: 744–752

Matrisan L M, Bowden G T, Krieg P et al 1986 The mRNA coding for the secreted protease transin is expressed more abundantly in malignant than in benign tumors. Proc Natl Acad Sci USA 83: 9413–9417

McKeehan W L, Adams P S, Fast D 1987 Different hormonal requirements for androgen-independent growth of normal and tumor epithelial cells from rat prostate. In Vitro Cell Dev Biol 23: 147–152

Meyers R M, Maniatis T, Lerman L S 1987 Detection and localization of single base changes by denaturing gradient gel electrophoresis. Methods Enzymol 155: 501–527

Mori H, Maki M, Oshi K et al 1990 Increased expression of genes for basic fibroblast growth factor and transforming growth factor type β–2 in human benign prostatic hyperplasia. Prostate 16: 71–80

Morris G L, Dodd J G 1990 Epidermal growth factor receptor mRNA levels in human prostatic tumors and cell lines. J Urol 143: 1272–1274

Myrdal S E, Twardzik D R, Auersperg N 1986 Cell-mediated co-action of transforming growth factors: incubation of type β with normal rat kidney cells produces a soluble activity that prolongs the ruffling response to type α. J Cell Biol 102: 1230–1234

Nicolson G L 1991 Quantitative variations in gene expression: possible role in cellular diversification and tumor progression. J Cell Biochem 46: 277–283

Orita M, Suzuki Y, Sekiya T et al 1989 Rapid and sensitive detection of point mutations and DNA polymorphisms using the polymerase chain reaction. Genomics 5: 874–879

Peehl D M, Wehner N, Stamey T A 1987 Activated Ki-*ras* oncogene in human prostatic adenocarcinoma. Prostate 10: 281–289

Perkel V S, Mohan S, Herring S J et al 1990 Human prostatic cancer cells, PC3, elaborate mitogenic activity which selectively stimulates human bone cells. Cancer Res 50: 6902–6907

Rijnders A W M, Van der Korput J A G M, Van Steenbrugge G J et al 1985 Expression of cellular oncogenes in human prostatic carcinoma cell lines. Biochem Biophys Res Commun 132: 548–554

Rizzinno A 1988 Transforming growth factor-β: multiple effects on cell differentiation and extracellular matrices. Dev Biol 130: 411–422

Roberts A B, Sporn M B, Assoian R K et al 1986 Transforming growth factor type β: rapid induction of fibrosis and angiogenesis *in vivo* and stimulation of collagen formation *in vitro* Proc Natl Acad Sci USA 83: 4167–4171

St Arnaud R, Poyet P, Walker P et al 1988 Androgens modulate epidermal growth factor receptor levels in the rat ventral prostate. Mol Cell Endocrinol 56: 21–27

Samowitz W S, Paull G, Hamilton S R 1988 Reported binding of monoclonal antibody RAP–5 to formalin-fixed tissue sections is not indicative of *ras* p21 expression. Hum Pathol 19: 127–132

Schalken J A, Ebeling S B, Isaacs J T et al 1988 Down modulation of fibronectin mRNA in metastizing rat prostatic cancer cells revealed by differential hybridization analysis. Cancer Res 48: 2042–2048

Starling J J, Sieg S M, Beckett M L et al 1986 Human prostate tissue antigens defined by murine monoclonal antibodies. Cancer Res 46: 367–374

Steeg P S, Bevilacqua G B, Kopper L et al 1988 Evidence for a novel gene associated with low tumor metastatic potential. J Natl Cancer Inst 80: 200–204

Sumiya H, Masai M, Akimoto S et al 1990 Histochemical examination of expression of ras p21 protein and R1881-binding protein in human prostatic cancers. Eur J Cancer 26: 786–789

Suzuki Y, Orita M, Shiraishi M et al 1990 Detection of ras gene mutations in human lung cancers by single-strand conformation analysis of polymerase chain reaction products. Oncogene 5: 1037–1043

Thompson T C 1990 Growth factors and oncogenes in prostate cancer. Cancer Cells 2: 345–354

Van der Kwast T H, Schalken J A, Ruizeveld-de Winter J A et al 1991 Androgen receptors in endocrine-therapy-resistant human prostate cancer. Int J Cancer 48: 189–193

Viola M V, Fromowitz F, Ovarez S et al 1986 Expression of *ras* oncogene p21 in prostate cancer. N Engl J Med 314: 133–137

Webb K S, Paulson D F, Parks S F et al 1984 Characterization of prostate tissue directed monoclonal antibody: alpha-Pro 13. Cancer Immunol Immunother 17: 7–17

Wilding G, Zugmeier G, Knabbe C et al 1989 Differential effects of transforming growth factor β on human prostate cancer cells *in vitro*. Mol Cell Endocrinol 62: 79–87

Wilson M J, Ditmanson J V, Sinha A A et al 1990 Plasminogen activator activities in the ventral and dorsolateral prostatic lobes of ageing Fischer 344 rats. Prostate 16: 147–161

5. Cytogenetics and molecular biology of testicular germ cell tumours

T. Strohmeyer   R. Ackermann

CYTOGENETIC STUDIES

Cytogenetic studies in human testicular germ cell tumours (GCT) indicate that these malignancies frequently contain gross genetic alterations. These include trisomy, breakage and loss of genetic material in the paracentromeric area of chromosome 1 (Wang et al 1980, Delozier-Blanchet et al 1985, Atkin & Baker 1985). Further alterations are translocation of 17q, which may also be present in multiple copies (Atkin & Baker 1983, Gibas et al 1986), and rearrangement of 6q, which has been found either deleted or translocated (Delozier-Blanchet et al 1987). GCT are generally hyperdiploid or hypertriploid with chromosome numbers between 60 and 69 in most seminomas and 50 to 59 in most teratomas (Atkin 1973).

In 1983 Atkin and Baker reported on an isochromosome of the short arm of chromosome 12, which was found in 4 seminomas and designated as i(12q). This finding was later confirmed by various groups (Gibas et al 1984, Delozier-Blanchet et al 1985, Bosl et al 1989, Castedo et al 1989). It was observed in seminomas as well as in non-seminomas. This observation is of particular interest since i(12p) has been detected in only 2 out of more than 3500 leukaemia specimens and in none of 600 lymphomas and 200 solid tumours other than GCT. Both leukaemia patients with i(12p) also had GCT (Bosl et al 1989). It is logical to assume that the high frequency of i(12p) may have useful clinical implications related to prognosis and diagnosis of GCT, as well as for the study of its tumorigenesis. In the same study, Bosl et al investigated 29 tumour specimens of 24 patients and observed i(12p) in 20 specimens of all primary sites and histologies of 16 of these patients. Furthermore, the study suggested that the copy number of i(12p) may be prognostically important, since the presence of three or more copies of i(12p) was associated with a higher risk of residual disease and treatment failure. All six patients with tumours containing three or more copies of i(12p) demonstrated some degree of resistance to initial systemic chemotherapy.

In addition, presence of i(12p) may be used in the classification of carcinomas with uncertain histology.

MOLECULAR BIOLOGY

The finding that 12p is the locus of the Ki-ras2 proto-oncogene led to speculations as to whether proto-oncogenes are involved in the process of malignant transformation in GCT.

A few studies on GCT have been conducted at the molecular level. In one immunohistochemical study increased expression of the c-myc protein, p62, was detected in 11 seminomas, whereas decreased expression was found in 21 malignant teratomas. A negative prognosis of the malignant teratomas was associated with the extent of decrease in c-myc expression in these tumours (Sikora et al 1985). Amplification and/or mRNA overexpression of the c-Ki-ras proto-oncogene was found in various testicular tumour cell lines and in 7 out of 10 metastases from testicular embryonal cell carcinomas (Wang et al 1987, Dmitrovsky et al 1990). However, in an immunohistochemical study performed on two primary GCT, the p21 ras-oncoprotein was not detected (Tanaka et al 1986). In another study, expression of the hst1 proto-oncogene was found in 5 out of 9 GCT including 2 seminomas (Yoshida et al 1988).

These findings have stimulated a more systematic analysis of a number of proto-oncogenes in a large cohort of GCT in order to establish a database that could be used to:

a. gain insights into initiation and/or progression of GCT
b. correlate molecular genetic findings with clinical parameters and survival
c. extend conventional tumour classifications
d. define high-risk patients with a potentially poor prognosis.

These studies focused on the proto-oncogenes c-kit, her–2/neu, hst1, int2, TGF-alpha, and the retinoblastoma tumour suppressor gene (RB) (Strohmeyer et al 1991a,b).

The findings on c-kit, hst1 and RB are of particular interest. C-kit is the cellular homologue of the viral oncogene (v-kit) of the feline sarcoma retrovirus HZ4–FeSV, encoding for an oncoprotein of 145 kd (Besmer et al 1986, Yarden et al 1987). The protein is a cell surface receptor with tyrosine kinase activity. Its ligand is the growth factor 'SCF' (stem cell factor) that is involved in the regulation of haematopoiesis and spermatogenesis (Zsebo et al 1990, Williams et al 1990, Huang et al 1990).

Hst1 is a cellular oncogene originally isolated from a human stomach carcinoma. The oncoprotein, with a molecular weight of 21 kd, is a fibroblast growth factor expressed in several embry onal tissues, but not in adult tissues (Delli-Bovi et al 1987, Yoshida et al 1988). Considering the embryonal component present in some histological types of GCT, investigation of this oncogene seemed particularly promising. Figure 5.1 shows a Northern blot analysis of the c-kit and hst1 mRNA expression in pairs of normal and malignant testicular tissues. The most striking observation is the inverse relationship between the expression of c-kit and hst1 in GCT. Hst1 is

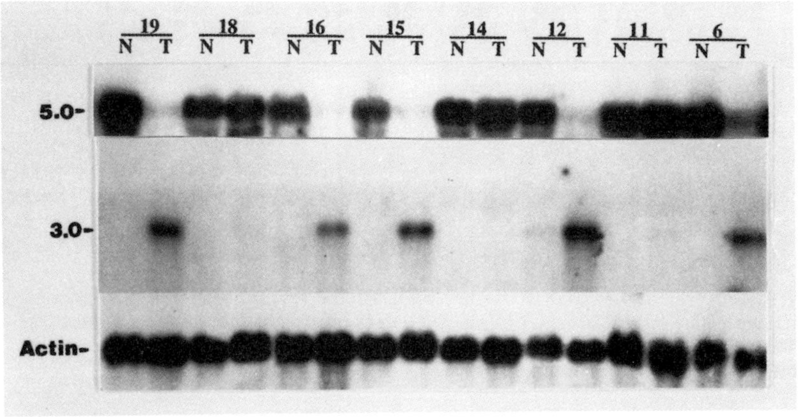

Fig. 5.1 Inverse relationship of hst1 (3.0 kb transcript)- and c-kit (5.0 kb transcript)-expression: Significant and equal c-kit expression in tumour and normal tissue of seminoma/normal pairs (pairs 11, 14) and in one mixed-tumour/normal pair comprised of vast areas of seminoma (pair 18). Absent or markedly decreased c-kit expression in the tumour tissue of non-seminoma/normal pairs (pairs 6, 12, 15, 16, 19). Hst1 is expressed in non-seminomas only (No. 6, 12, 15, 16, 19) and tumour tissues expressing hst1 do not express high levels of c-kit. (The faint hst1 signal seen in sample 12N is likely to be due to minor microscopic invasive tumour infiltration found at the border of this specimen.) (Reproduced with kind permission from Strohmeyer et al 1991a.)

almost exclusively expressed in non-seminomatous tumour tissues, whereas c-kit is expressed in normal testicular tissues and most seminomas. Absent or decreased c-kit expression is observed in almost all non-seminomas. The study has also demonstrated that the expression of c-kit in normal testicular tissues depends on the presence of an intact spermatogenesis. C-kit expression is decreased or absent in testes with altered spermatogenesis, as is frequently found in cryptorchic or atrophic testes. The c-kit gene has been determined to be allelic with the dominant so-called 'white spotting locus' of the mouse. Mutations of this locus not only affect murine haematopoiesis but inhibit the proliferation and migration of primordial germ cells during mouse development (Chabot et al 1988, Geissler et al 1988). In the light of this phenomenon, c-kit may be a relevant factor in the tumorigenesis of seminomas as well as in normal human spermatogenesis, especially since the ligand of c-kit, stem cell factor, has recently been shown to be expressed at RNA and protein level in normal human testicular tissues (Strohmeyer et al 1992). Furthermore, alterations of structure or expression of these genes in otherwise normal testicular tissue may be of importance in various infertility states.

The retinoblastoma tumour suppressor gene (RB), first discovered in retinoblastomas, is again of particular interest since the biological features of retinoblastomas have some similarities with GCT. The question is, whether

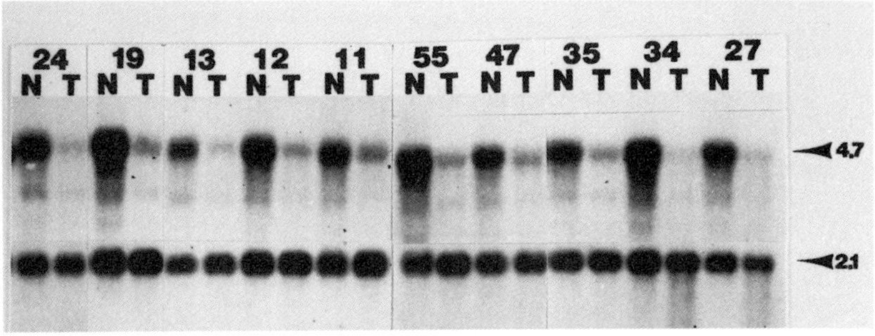

Fig. 5.2 Northern-blot analysis of the retinoblastoma gene RNA. There is distinct reduction of the RB-mRNA (4.7 kb) in the tissues of malignant germ cell tumours of various histologies (T) and expression in macroscopically normal adjacent testicular tissues (N). The 2.1-kb transcript is β-actin.

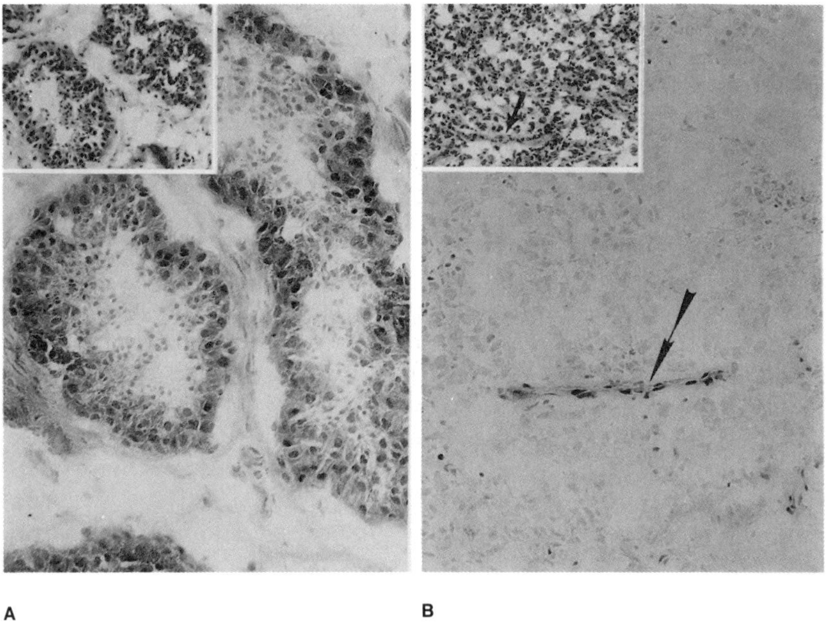

Fig. 5.3 Immunohistochemical analysis of the expression of the RB-encoded nuclear protein. **A** Normal testicular tissue with preserved seminiferous tubules (×320). Positive staining of nuclei of spermatogonia, spermatocytes and Sertoli cells. Heterogeneous staining pattern in the more mature spermatids and spermatozoas. Inset: Haematoxylin/eosin (HE)-staining of a serial section of the same area (×160). **B** Seminoma germ cell tumour (×320). There is no nuclear staining in the tumour cells, whereas strong nuclear staining occurs in endothelial cells (arrow) and lymphocytes found in the section. Inset: Haematoxylin/eosin (HE)-staining of a serial section of the same area (×160).

GCT demonstrates alterations of the structure or expression of RB. The ubiquitously expressed RB-protein is believed to function as a cell cycle regulator whose active form keeps cells in the G0–G1 phase of the cell cycle (DeCaprio et al 1988, 1989, Buchkovich et al 1989, Lee et al 1987, Whyte et al 1988). Northern blot analysis of RB demonstrates a distinct reduction of RB mRNA in tissues of malignant GCT as compared to the expression in normal adjacent testicular tissues (Fig. 5.2). Immunohistochemical analysis of the expression of the RB-encoded nuclear protein in normal testis shows staining in nuclei of spermatogonia, spermatocytes and Sertoli cells, and a heterogenous staining pattern in the more mature spermatids and spermatozoas. No nuclear staining of the tumour cells could be demonstrated in seminomas and most non-seminomas (Fig. 5.3). Immunohistochemical analysis of teratocarcinomas, however, demonstrated a heterogenous staining pattern: differentiated tumour cells mimicking mature cellular components such as epithelium or cartilage showed intensive staining, whereas undifferentiated tumour cells were not stained (Fig. 5.4). In sections of specimens in which the adjacent macroscopically normal tissue contained carcinoma in situ (CIS), no RB protein could be detected in the CIS cells. No alterations have been detected at the DNA level by Southern blot analysis in any of the tumours. However, this technique may not be sensitive enough to reveal minor lesions or point mutations.

The relevance of the observation that all GCT, both seminomas and

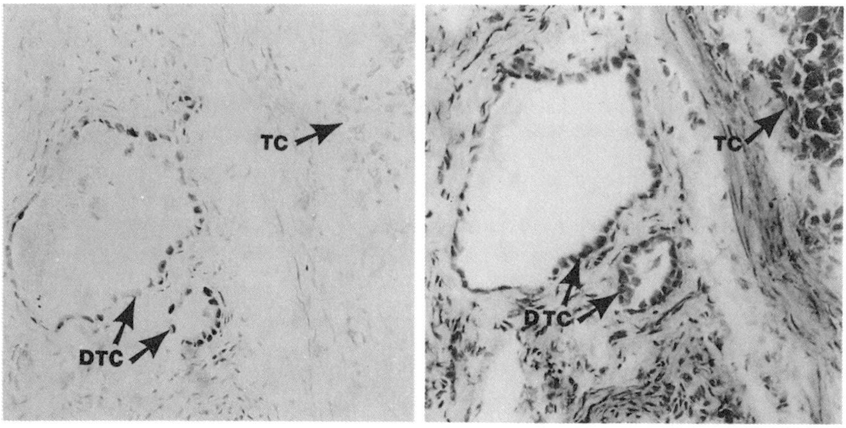

A B

Fig. 5.4 **A** Immunohistochemical analysis of the RB-encoded protein (×20). This is a non-seminoma germ cell tumour (teratocarcinoma subtype). Hetereogeneous protein expression was found in the tumour. Differentiated tumour cells (DTC) mimicking mature epithelium show positive nuclear staining, while the less differentiated tumour cells (TC) do not stain. **B** Haematoxylin/eosin (HE)-staining of a serial section of the same area (×20).

non-seminomas, lack expression of RB protein (except in differentiated teratoma cells) is unclear. The precise contribution of changes in RB expression to the pathogenesis of human GCT remains to be determined. It is unlikely, however, that decreased RB expression is the only event responsible for the development of GCT, since these tumours rarely develop as a secondary malignancy in patients with inherited retinoblastoma.

SUMMARY

Chromosomal alterations, oncogene alterations and changes of RB-suppressor gene expression are frequently detectable in testicular GCT. Modern molecular genetic techniques are certainly suitable to further investigate the pathogenic significance of these findings and their relevance for diagnosis and therapy of human germ cell tumours.

REFERENCES

Atkin N B 1973 High chromosome numbers of seminomata and malignant teratomata of the testis: a review of data on 103 tumours. Br J Cancer 28: 275–279

Atkin N B, Baker M C 1983 i(12p): specific chromosomal marker in seminoma and malignant teratoma of the testis? Cancer Genet Cytogenet 10: 199–204

Atkin N B, Baker M C 1985 Chromosome analysis of three seminomas. Cancer Genet Cytogenet 17: 315–323

Besmer P, Murphy J E, George P C et al 1986 A new acute transforming feline retrovirus and relationship of its oncogene v-kit with the protein kinase gene family. Nature 320: 415–421

Bosl G J, Dmitrovsky E, Reuter V E et al 1989 Isochromosome of chromosome 12: Clinically useful marker for male germ cell tumors. JNCI 81: 1874–1878

Buchkovich K, Duffy L A, Harlow E 1989 The retinoblastoma protein is phosphorylated during specific phases of the cell cycle. Cell 58: 1097–1105

Castedo S M M J, de Jong B, Oosterhuis J W 1989 Cytogenetic analysis of ten human seminomas. Cancer Res 49: 439–443

Chabot B, Stephenson D A, Chapman V M 1988 The proto-oncogene c-kit encoding a transmembrane tyrosine kinase receptor maps to the mouse W locus. Nature 335: 88–89

DeCaprio J A, Ludlow J W, Figge J 1988 SV 40 large tumor antigen forms a specific complex with the product of the retinoblastoma susceptibility gene. Cell 54: 275–283

DeCaprio J A, Ludlow J W, Lynch D 1989 The product of the retinoblastoma susceptibility gene has properties of a cell cycle regulatory element. Cell 58: 1085–1095

Delli-Bovi P, Curatola A M, Kern 1987 An oncogene isolated by transfection of Kaposi's sarcoma DNA encodes a growth factor that is a member of the FGF family. Cell 50: 729–737

Delozier-Blanchet C D, Engel E, Walt H 1985 Isochromosome 12p in malignant testicular tumours. Cancer Genet Cytogenet 15: 375–376

Delozier-Blanchet C D, Walt H, Engel E et al 1987 Cytogenetic studies of human testicular germ cell tumours. Int J Androl 1: 69–77

Dmitrovsky E, Murty V V V, Moy D 1990 Isochromosome 12p, i(12p), in male germ cell tumour (GCT) cell line: karyologic amplification of ki-ras2 without point-mutational activation. Proc Am Assoc Cancer Res 31: 27 (Abstract No. 156)

Geissler E N, Ryan M A, Housman D E 1988 The dominant-white spotting (W) locus of the mouse encodes the c-kit proto-oncogene. Cell 55: 185–192

Gibas Z, Prout G R Jr, Sandberg A A 1984 Malignant teratoma of the testis with an isochromosome No. 12, i(12p), as the sole structural cytogenetic abnormality. J Urol 131: 762–763

Gibas Z, Prout G R Jr, Pontes J E 1986 Chromosome changes in germ cell tumours of the testis. Cancer Genet Cytogenet 19: 245–252

Huang E, Nocka K, Beier D R 1990 The hematopoietic growth factor KL is encoded by the SI locus and is the ligand of the c-kit receptor, the gene product of the W locus. Cell 63: 225–233
Lee W-H, Shew J-Y, Hong F D 1987 The retinoblastoma susceptibility gene encodes a nuclear phosphoprotein associated with DNA binding activity. Nature 329: 642–645
Sikora K, Evan G, Stewart J 1985 Detection of the myc-oncogene product in testicular cancer. Br J Cancer 52: 171–176
Strohmeyer T, Peter S, Hartmann M 1991a Expression of the hst-1 and c-kit protooncogenes in human testicular germ cell tumors. Cancer Res 51: 1811–1816
Strohmeyer T, Reissmann P, Cordon-Cardo C 1991b Correlation between retinoblastoma gene expression and differentiation in human testicular tumors. Proc Natl Acad Sci (USA) 88: 6662–6666
Strohmeyer T, Reese D, Zsebo K 1992 Expression of the c-kit proto-oncogene and its ligand 'stem cell factor (SCF)' in normal and malignant human and testicular tissue: potential involvement in spermatogenesis and oncogenesis. (In preparation)
Tanaka T, Slamon D J, Battifora H 1986 Expression of p21 ras oncoproteins in human cancers. Cancer Res 46: 1465–1470
Wang L, Vass W, Gao C 1987 Amplification and enhanced expression of the c-Ki-ras2 protooncogene in human embryonal carcinomas. Cancer Res 46: 4192–4198
Wang N, Trend B, Bronson D L 1980 Nonrandom abnormalities in chromosome 1 in human testicular cancers. Cancer Res 40: 796–802
Whyte P, Buchkovich K J, Horowitz J M 1988 Association between an oncogene and an anti-oncogene: the adenovirus E1A proteins bind to the retinoblastoma gene product. Nature 334: 124–128
Williams D E, Eisenman J, Baird A 1990 Identification of a ligand for the c-kit proto-oncogene. Cell 63: 167–174
Yarden Y, Kuang W-J, Yang-Feng T 1987 Human proto-oncogene c-kit: a new cell surface receptor tyrosine kinase for an unidentified ligand. EMBO J. 6: 3341–3351
Yoshida T, Tsutsumi M, Sakamoto H 1988 Expression of the HST1 oncogene in human germ cell tumors (Published erratum appears in Biochem. Biophys Res. Comm. 157: 850, 1988). Biochem Biophys Res Comm 155: 1324–9
Zsebo K M, Williams D A, Geissler E N 1990 Stem cell factor is encoded at the SI locus of the mouse and is the ligand for the c-kit tyrosine kinase receptor. Cell 63: 213–224

6. Specific detection of metastasized human tumour cells in embryonic chicks by the polymerase chain reaction

T. Uchibayashi H. Hisazumi K. Kazuto T. Hasegawa Y. Endo M. Noguchi T. Sasaki

INTRODUCTION

In cancer treatment, the extent of infiltration of the cancer and the presence of metastases are known to be important factors influencing the prognosis of the patient. When the primary focus is discovered at an early stage, local radical treatment may be feasible by means of surgical resection, radiotherapy, hyperthermia, and chemotherapy as well as combination therapy using two or more of these modalities. However, when the primary tumour has assumed a certain size, systemic micrometastases are assumed to be present, and chemotherapy, immunotherapy, and whole body hyperthermia are usually resorted to at this stage. In addition, it is well recognized that the sensitivity of metastatic and primary cancer cells to anti-cancer agents differs appreciably. Thus, it is thought that knowledge prior to the initiation of treatment of the sensitivity of metastatic tumours to various drugs as well as hyperthermia would greatly contribute to enhancing the therapeutic results when radical treatment is being attempted.

Most hitherto conducted research on metastases has focused on elucidation of the mechanisms involved in the metastatic process. In contrast, little attention has been directed to therapeutic approaches to metastatic cancer cells, possibly because few effective experimental metastasis models have been established. The nude mouse has been the most frequently used host in xenograft experiments, although this metastasis model suffers from several drawbacks including; 1) a low rate of successful tumour implantation; 2) the necessity for special pathogen-free facilities to raise the animals; 3) long waiting period before results are obtained; and 4) an extremely low rate of metastasis formation. In the present study, we used the chick embryonic assay, which is both simple and inexpensive to perform and in which a high rate of tumour implantation is achieved, to detect metastatic tumours and to quantify the sensitivity of metastatic tumours to various forms of therapy (Karnofsky et al 1952, Ossowski et al 1980, Sherbet et al 1980,

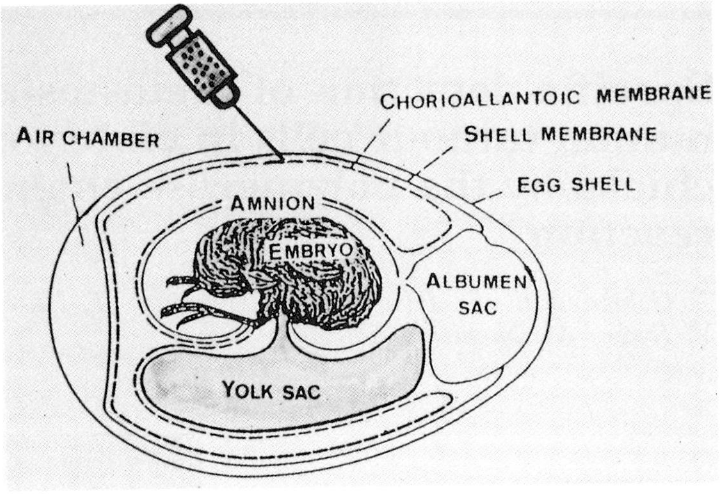

Fig. 6.1 Diagram of a fertilized egg.

Chambers et al 1982, Nishikawa et al 1987). This chick embryonic assay has not been entirely satisfactory as a quantitative metastasis experimental model because, due to the short experimental period of seven days, the number of tumour cells in the developing metastatic foci is extremely small, and so detection of metastatic foci has depended on the histopathological findings. Recently, the polymerase chain reaction (PCR) technique has been developed for highly sensitive detection by amplifying a small segment of DNA flanked by oligonucleotide primers of known DNA sequences

A

a Huβ-1: 5′-AGAGCCATCTATTGCTTACA-3′
b Huβ-8 5′-TATGACATGAACTTAACCAT-3′
c Huβ-2: 5′ACACAACTGTGTTCACTAGC-3′

B

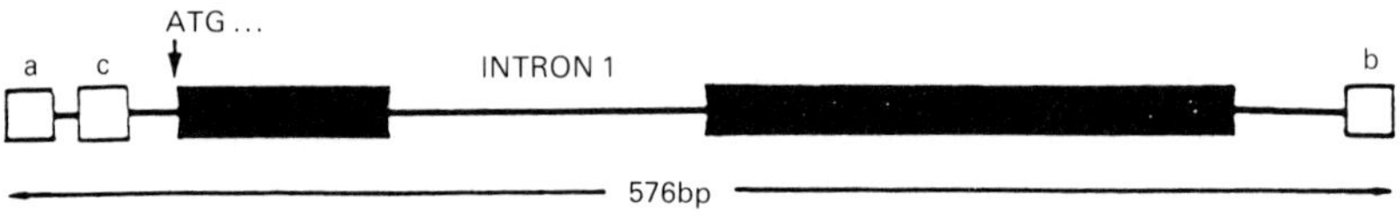

Fig. 6.2 Oligonucleotide primers and probe for PCR amplification and their locations in human β-globin gene **A** Sequences of oligonucleotide primers and probe used in PCR. **B** Location of the oligonucleotides.

(Saiki et al 1985). In the present study, using the PCR we amplified a specific human tumour cell-derived DNA sequence present in embryonic chick organ metastases and analyzed it by Southern blotting.

METHODS AND RESULTS

This method will be explained in brief. Figure 6.1 shows a diagram of a fertilized egg. Lying just beneath the shell is the shell membrane, below which is found the chorioallantoic membrane. This chorioallantoic membrane, which is made up of partially adhering chorionic epithelium and allantoic epithelium, extends beneath the shell membrane. Blood vessels developing between these membranes play an important role in the respiration of the embryo. In metastasis experiments using the chick embryonic assay, either tumours are placed onto the chorioallantoic membrane of 10-day fertilized eggs, or tumour cells are injected into chorioallantoic membrane veins. Seven days later, on the 17th day of embryonic life, the liver and lungs of the embryo are dissected, and the DNA of each organ is extracted using a rapid DNA preparation method (Davis et al 1986). Next, 1 mg of DNA as a template is amplified by 25 cycles of PCR, during which double-stranded DNA is denatured, primers are added, and complementary strands synthesized, resulting in approximately 100 000-fold amplification of the target DNA fragment. The amplified DNA fragments are then analyzed by Southern blotting.

In the present study, a portion of the β-globin gene was selected as the human DNA-specific target for amplification, and from a DNA sequence of this gene primers and a probe were prepared for PCR. Figure 6.2 shows the DNA sequence of the human β-globin gene. For the metastasis experiments, Hub-1 and Hub-8 which flank the first and second exons were selected as the PCR primers. The length of the DNA fragment amplified by PCR was 576 bp. The Hub-2 shown in Figure 6.2 was labelled with ^{32}P and used as the probe. Human fibrosarcoma HT-1080 cells (Rasheed et al 1974), which are known to metastasize spontaneously in nude mice, were injected into the veins of 10-day embryos, and the metastasis-bearing organs dissected seven days later. Figure 6.3 shows the results of PCR performed in the samples after DNA extraction. As expected, no PCR-amplified products were detected in the DNA derived from the organs of the control chick embryos, while in the tumour cell-inoculated embryonic liver, amplification bands were detected by autoradiography in proportion to the number of HT-1080 cells implanted (1×10^3–1×10^6cells). These results demonstrate that the quantitative and specific detection of human tumour metastatic cells present in the organs of chick embryos is possible with this method.

Next, HT-1080 DNA was serially diluted with embryonic liver DNA and subjected to PCR amplification. As seen in Figure 6.4, detection of DNA of HT-1080 origin was feasible when quantities as small as 0.1 ng (0.01% of

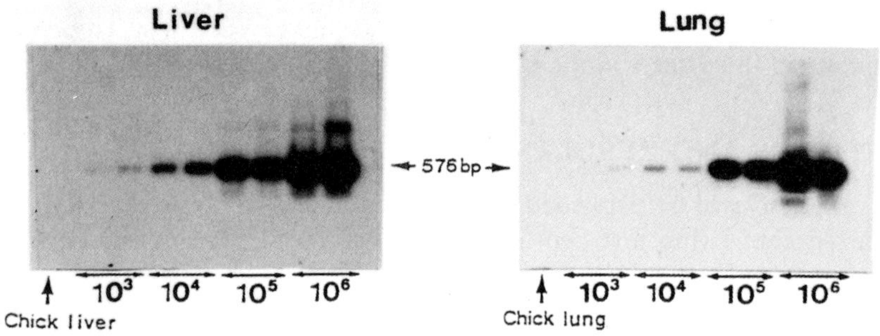

Fig. 6.3 Detection of metastasis in embryonic liver and lung following intravenous injection of HT-1080 cells.

the total) were present. Growth kinetics in the embryonic liver over time were then studied. Figure 6.5 shows the results obtained by injecting HT-1080 and human fibroblast KMST-6 cells (Namba et al 1985) into the chorioallantoic membrane veins and amplifying the extracted DNA by PCR. The amplified DNA fragments from the HT-1080 cells showed a

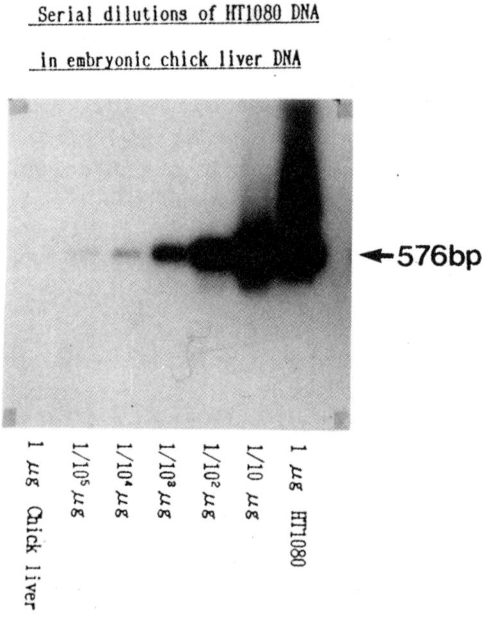

Fig. 6.4 Southern analysis of PCR amplification products of the human β-globin gene.

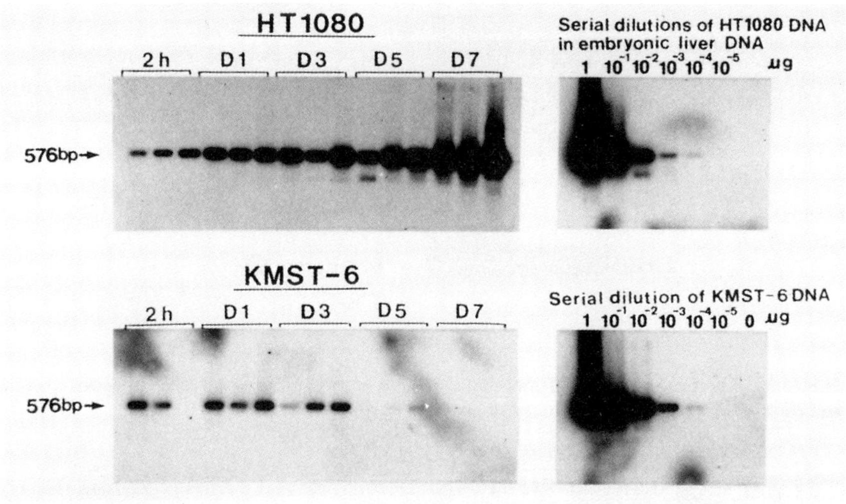

Fig. 6.5 Kinetics of growth of metastatic cells in embryonic liver after intravenous injection of HT-1080 and human fibroblast KMST-6 cells (10^6 cells/embryo).

gradual increase from 2 hours to 7 days after inoculation, suggesting that the metastatic cells proliferated in the embryonic liver. On the other hand, with the KMST-6 cells, amplified DNA fragments were seen from 2 hours until 3 days after inoculation, but showed a sharp decrease from the 5th day with almost no PCR products detectable by the 7th day. Changes over time in the number of metastatic cells are shown in the graph found in Figure 6.6.

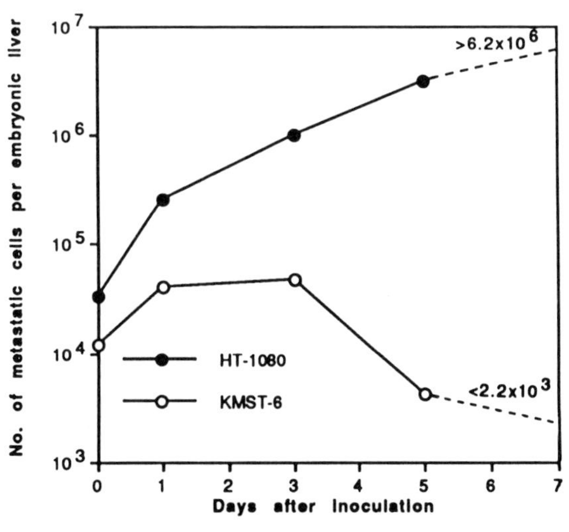

Fig. 6.6 Kinetics of growth of metastatic cells in embryonic liver.

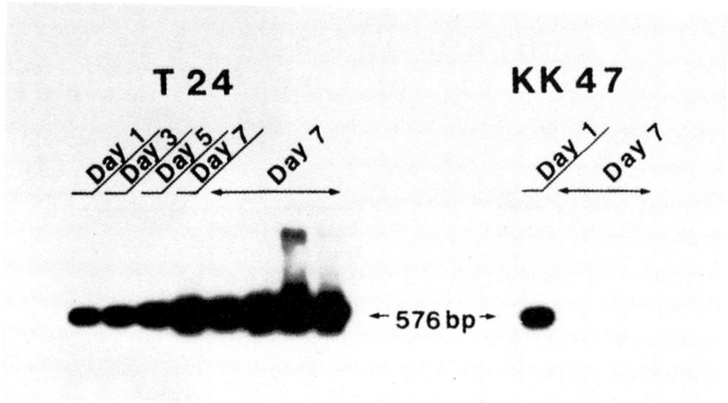

Fig. 6.7 Kinetics of growth of metastatic cells in embryonic liver after intravenous injection of T-24 and KK-47 cells (10^6 cells/embryo).

It was suggested that the HT-1080 cell-derived DNA was not merely trapped in the liver, but that after metastasizing to the liver cell proliferation occurred. Conversely, in the case of fibroblast KMST-6 cells, although the inoculated cells themselves were transiently trapped in the liver, these cells were subsequently unable to proliferate.

Using the same techniques, cultured urinary bladder cancer-derived cell line T-24 (kindly supplied by Prof. V. Peter Collins, Sahlgrenska Hospital, Gothenburg) and KK-47 cells (Taya et al 1977) were implanted into chick embryos, and the presence of metastatic cells in the liver determined. As shown in Figure 6.7, like HT-1080, the T-24 cells showed metastatic cell proliferation with time. In contrast, in the case of the KK-47 cells, no metastatic cell proliferation was found.

Treatment experiments using adriamycin to the metastatic foci formed by this method were then carried out. Either 1×10^5 or 1×10^6 HT-1080

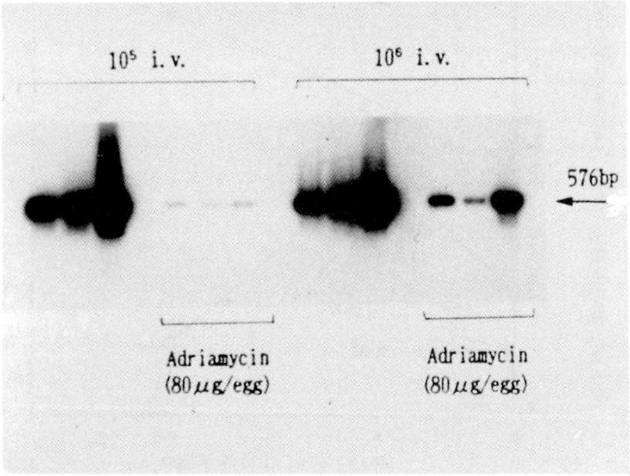

Fig. 6.8 Effect of adriamycin on liver metastasis of HT-1080 cells in embryonic chick.

Table 6.1 Effect of adriamycin (ADM) on liver metastasis of HT-1080 cells in the embryonic chick*

Number of cells injected	Drug	Dose (μg/egg)	Radioactivity (AU/mm^2) ± SD	Inhibition ratio (%)
1 × 10^6	ADM	80	62.5 ± 53.9	88.2
	Control		527.6 ± 458.7	
1 × 10^5	ADM	80	5.2 ± 1.5	98.9
	Control		486.5 ± 252.3	

*HT-1080 cells were injected into chorioallantoic membrane (CAM) vein of 11–day embryo. ADM was injected into the CAM vein 3 days later.

tumour cells were inoculated into the chorioallantoic membrane veins of chick embryos, 3 days after which 80 μg/egg of adriamycin were administered intravenously. On the 7th day after inoculation the embryonic liver was dissected, the extracted DNA amplified by PCR, and the presence of metastatic cells examined. Administration of adriamycin alone resulted in a clear decrease in the amount of PCR-amplified DNA (Fig. 6.8). The radioactivity of these bands was analyzed and compared in the groups administered and not administered adriamycin (Table 6.1). Inoculated cell proliferation inhibition rates of 88.2% and 98.9% were achieved in the former when 1 × 10^6 and 1 × 10^5 cells respectively were inoculated, suggesting that HT-1080 cells are sensitive to adriamycin. Chemosensitivity tests were conducted in the same fashion using other agents as well. Findings suggesting an inhibitory effect on metastases were obtained, with decreases in bands attained with adriamycin, vinblastin, and cyclophosphamide in decreasing order of effect (Fig. 6.9). When the radioactivity of the PCR products was compared with that of the control group, decreases of 93.8% with adriamycin 80 μg/egg, 86.6% with vinblastin 1 μg/egg, and 76.3% with cyclophosphamide 500 μg/egg were found. In contrast, no tumour proliferation inhibitory effect was found with CDDP administration (Table 6.2).

Table 6.2 Effect of anti-tumour drugs on liver metastasis of HT-1080 cells in the embryonic chick*

Drug	Dose (μg/egg)	Radioactivity (AU/mm^2) ± SD	Inhibition ratio (%)
CPM	240	209.6 ± 137.5	4.6
	500	52.0 ± 18.9	76.3
CDDP	5	207.6 ± 46.0	5.3
	10	219.7 ± 80.0	−0.2
ADM	40	23.0 ± 13.2	89.5
	80	13.7 ± 9.4	93.8
VBL	0.5	98.4 ± 50.0	55.1
	1	29.3 ± 31.5	86.6
Control		219.2 ± 128.2	

*HT-1080 cells (1 × 10^5 cells) were injected into chorioallantoic membrane (CAM) vein of 11-day embryo.
Drugs were injected into the CAM vein 3 days later.

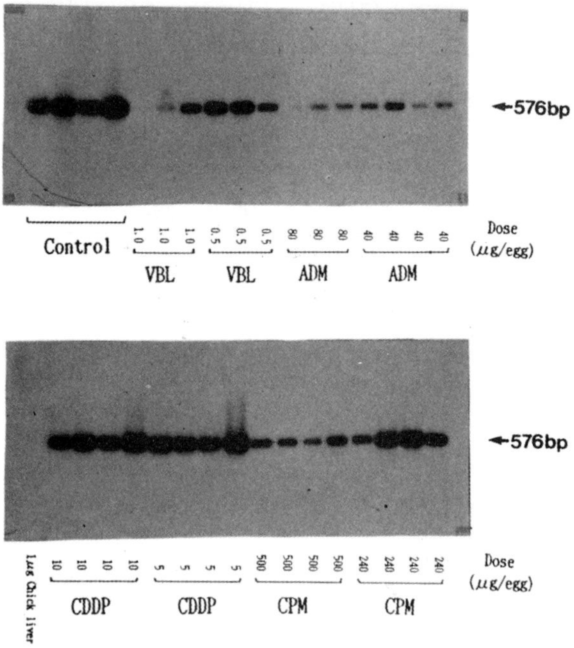

Fig. 6.9 Effect of antitumour drugs on liver metastasis of HT-1080 cells in embryonic chick.

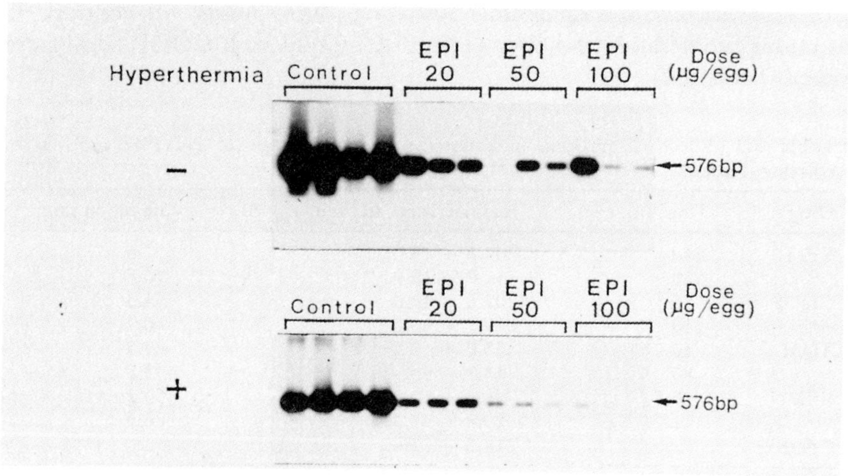

Fig. 6.10 Inhibitory effect of epirubicin with/without hyperthermia on liver metastasis of HT-1080 cells in the embryonic chick.

The anti-tumour effect of the adriamycin derivative epirubicin by itself or in combination with hyperthermia was then studied. An even greater decrease in the amount of PCR-products was seen when this agent was combined with hyperthermia, with findings suggesting an enhancement of the effect of combined hyperthermia for metastatic foci (Fig. 6.10). Although further examination of the optimal drug concentration is thought to be necessary, when the radioactivity values were determined, a metastatic cell proliferation inhibitory effect was found with epirubicin administration alone, and was further enhanced when hyperthermia was used in combination.

SUMMARY

In DNA samples obtained from the organs of chick embryos inoculated with human tumour cells, PCR was used to amplify a DNA fragment specific to the human β-globin gene. By detecting these amplified DNA fragments, the feasibility of efficiently detecting metastatic cells present in chick embryos was demonstrated.

This method is an excellent quantitative experimental metastasis model and holds considerable promise as a screening method that may provide useful information about the human tumour metastasis inhibitory effect of various anti-cancer agents and hyperthermia.

REFERENCES

Chambers A F, Shafir R, Ling V 1982 A model system for studying metastasis using the embryonic chick. Cancer Res 42: 4018–4025

Davis L G, Dibner M D, Battey J F 1986 Basic methods in molecular biology. Elsevier Science Publishing, New York. pp 42–43

Karnofsky D A, Ridgway L P, Patterson P A 1952 Tumor transplantation to the chick embryo. Ann N Y Acad Sci 55: 313–329

Namba M, Nishitani K, Hydoh F et al 1985 Neoplastic transformation of human diploid fibroblasts (KMST-6) by treatment with ^{60}Co gamma rays. Int J Cancer 35: 275–280

Nishikawa K, Sasaki T, Tanaka M 1987 Experimental model for predicting metastatic ability of tumors using chick embryo. Jpn J Clin Oncol 17: 319–325

Ossowski L, Reich E 1980 Experimental model for quantitative study of metastasis. Cancer Res 40: 2300–2309

Rasheed S, Nelson-Rees W A, Toth E M et al 1974 Characterization of a newly derived human sarcoma cell line (HT-1080). Cancer 33: 1027–1033

Saiki R, Scharf S, Faloona F et al 1985 Enzymatic amplification of β-globin genomic sequences and restriction site analysis for diagnosis of sickle cell anemia. Science 230: 1350–1354

Sherbet G V, Lakshmi M S, Guy D A 1980 A possibility of predicting metastatic ability of tumours by implantation into chick embryos. Epigenetic grading of metastasizing and non-metastasizing forms of a hamster lymphosarcoma. Eur J Cancer 6: 561–568

Taya T, Kobayashi T, Tsukahara K et al 1977 In vitro culture of malignant tumor tissues from the human urinary tract. Jpn J Urol 11: 1003–1011

7. Cytogenetic abnormalities in renal cell carcinoma

A. V. Bono R. Casalone P. Granata

INTRODUCTION

It is well known that in familial renal cell carcinoma (RCC) chromosomal abnormalities, such as chromosome 3;11 translocation, can frequently be demonstrated. The expanding cytogenetic analysis in sporadic RCC has identified various chromosomal abnormalities, considering dominant either the translocation of the short arm of chromosome 3 or trisomy/tetrasomy of chromosome 7.

Some recent reports have suggested a possible correlation between the invasiveness of human tumours and genetic material located on chromosome 7 (Collard et al 1987); this is because the epidermal growth factor gene is located on chromosome 7 (Koprowsi et al 1985). In RCC, rearrangements of chromosome 3 in conjunction with trisomy 7 have been associated with higher stages and aggressive evolution (Weaver et al 1988), but other reports failed to confirm that these chromosome patterns may have prognostic significance (Teyssier & Ferre 1990, Ljungberg et al 1991).

As in the Varese district of Northern Italy the prevalence of RCC is particularly high (11.3 per 100 000), an integrated program of clinical research on RCC (search for/of disease, possible patient heavy metal exposure, immunochemistry on pathology specimens) is ongoing in Varese General Hospital. In this paper we report data on the cytogenetic analysis performed on kidney specimens of 64 consecutive patients affected by RCC.

MATERIALS AND METHODS

Between January 1989 and September 1991 cytogenetic analysis was performed on 64 patients (43 M, 21 F) affected by histologically confirmed RCC. Immediately after the nephrectomy the tissue fragments, belonging to areas of vital appearing tumour, were cut aseptically from the removed kidney.

Part of the specimen was washed into Ham's F–10 Medium containing antibiotics (penicillin and streptomycin) and 20% fetal calf serum, and minced with a sharp blade. The fragments were put in culture medium

RPMI 1640, which was substituted every three days, and incubated in 5% CO_2 at 37°C. When a growth occurred around the fragments, these were removed by a Pasteur's pipette and transferred to a new container. The remaining cells were cultured until an almost confluent growth rich in mitoses was observed. Then 0.01 μg/ml of Colcemid was added to the culture medium and cells removed using a trypsin solution (EDTA 0.1%). A hypotonic shock (0.75 M KCl) was applied for 7 minutes to the cells which were finally fixed in a 3:1 solution of methanol and acetic acid.

The second part of the specimen was subjected to proteolysis, by treatment with 0.8% Collagenase IA dissolved in RPMI 1640 for 12–48 hours. Cells suspended in the medium were then washed by 7 minutes centrifugation (1200 r.p.m.), resuspended in a new container (with three glass slides adhering to the bottom) with fresh RPMI 1640, and cultured at 37°C in 5% CO_2 for 7–9 days. The vital cells adhering to the bottom slides and giving a confluent growth were submitted to hypotonic shock and fixed as described above.

The banding technique for QFQ bands was employed and the modal number of chromosomes was determined after counting at least 25 metaphases. Numerical chromosome abnormalities were defined as clonal when the same anomaly was present in at least 2 metaphases. The constitutional karyotype was controlled on T lymphocytes stimulated by PHA.

RESULTS

In all 64 specimens the RCC was pathologically confirmed at the time of nephrectomy. The stage distribution was as follows: Stage I, 36 patients; Stage II, 8; Stage III, 14; Stage IV, 6 (Robson et al 1969). The mean follow-up at a cut off performed on September 1991 was 15 months (minimum 2, maximum 32). Clear cell carcinoma was present in 57 cases, granular cell carcinoma in 4 and sarcomatous patterns were found in 3.

The tissue culture was performed on all tumour samples and on 54 samples of normal tissue from the kidney bearing the tumour. Table 7.1 shows the results of cytogenetic analysis for the whole series.

In 34 tumoral cultures the chromosome analysis failed for the following reasons: absence of cellular growths: 16; no representative mitoses: 16; contamination: 2. Of the normal kidney cultures, 31 failed due to: absence of cellular growths, 12; no representative mitoses, 17; contamination, 2. Therefore only 30 tumoral cases and 23 normal kidney cases were considered suitable for the study.

In normal kidney tissue, chromosomal abnormalities were found in 11 of the 23 cases (47.8%). The main abnormality was the loss of the Y chromosome (7 cases); this was quite often associated with other abnormalities. Trisomy 7 and 10 were also frequently present – in 8 cases (34.7%) and 4 cases (17%), respectively.

In 20 of 30 (66%) tumours a variety of abnormalities were found and,

Table 7.1 Chromosomal abnormalities in normal kidneys and tumours related to the pathological stage of the disease

Patient		Tumour	Chromosomal abnormalities		No. of mitoses
Sex	Age	stage	Normal kidney	Tumour	in tumour tissue
M	64	I	Not done	−Y, +10	10
M	67	III	Not done	None	20
M	42	I	Not done	None	33
F	55	I	Not done	None	20
F	57	I	Not done	None	25
M	77	IV	Not done	−Y, del(1)(q32)	59
F	50	I	Not done	None	23
M	57	II	Not done	No growth	
M	70	II	Not done	No mitoses	
M	64	I	Not done	No growth	
F	45	I	None	No growth	
M	72	I	No mitoses	No mitoses	
M	56	IV	No growth	−Y	13
F	72	I	No growth	Contamination	
F	69	II	No growth	No growth	
F	53	I	None	+7, +17	20
M	64	I	No growth	No growth	
F	35	I	No growth	del(3)(p21–pter)	10
M	65	IV	No growth	−Y, +7	14
M	68	I	No mitoses	No growth	
M	67	I	None	None	10
M	58	I	−Y, +7	−Y	23
M	74	II	No growth	No mitoses	
F	67	III	No mitoses	No growth	
M	70	I	None	No mitoses	
F	67	IV	None	+(1:16)(q22–24)	15
M	66	I	No mitoses	−Y, t(13q;14q) +7 t(1;y)(q44;q12), t(4:6)(q21;q35), +2	27
M	58	I	No growth	No mitoses	
M	40	I	No growth	No growth	
M	56	IV	No growth	No growth	
M	54	III	−Y	−Y	45
M	69	III	No mitoses	No mitoses	
M	65	I	+7, +10	−Y, +7, +10, +13	12
M	69	III	−Y	No mitoses	
M	60	IV	;X, −Y, +del(Y), +7 +10, +15, +16, inv (2) (p25ql4) +9, +14	60–70, −y, +2, del (1)(lqter-cen-p11::?)	3
M	69	III	No mitoses	−Y	12
M	60	I	No mitoses	No growth	
M	36	I	46XY?	None	15
M	59	I	No mitoses	No growth	
M	58	I	No growth	No growth	
F	73	I	No mitoses	No mitoses	
M	34	III	No mitoses	No mitoses	
F	74	I	Contamination	Contamination	
F	39	III	None	None	20
F	63	II	del(6)(q23) del(4)(4qter-cen-p14), +7, +2del(1)(q32)	+10, +7, −13 48XXX, t(7;11) (q32;q14) inv (1)(q22;q36) t(1;8)(q23;q32) t(4;14)(q23;q31)	58

Table 7.1 (Contd.)

Patient		Tumour	Chromosomal abnormalities		No. of mitoses
Sex	Age	stage	Normal kidney	Tumour	in tumour tissue
F	63	III	No mitoses	60–90	30
M	59	II	−Y, +21, +7	No growth	
F	68	I	None	del(3)(p13)	5
F	46	I	+7, +10	52XX, +2, +5, +7, +14, +16, del(3), t(3;?)(qter-p24::?)	14
M	66	I	No growth	No growth	
M	75	I	No mitoses	No mitoses	
M	51	I	No mitoses	No mitoses	
F	46	III	−21, +10, +8	+7, +21, +10, 92XXXX, del(3) (q21)	27
M	63	III	+7, −Y, +13, +3	No growth	
M	56	I	None	−Y, −3, +21	5
M	63	III	del(Y)(q11), +7 +21	del(Y)(q11)	24
M	53	II	None	None	50
M	70	IV	No mitoses	No mitoses	
F	66	III	No mitoses	No mitoses	
M	53	III	None	None	2
M	69	III	None	No mitoses	
M	72	II	None	No mitoses	
F	60	I	None	None	7
F	45	I	No growth	No growth	

again, the loss of Y, and trisomies 7 and 10 were the most frequent. Deletion of the short arm of chromosome 3 and various translocations were also detectable.

In a significant number of cases (8) similar chromosomal abnormalities were found in both renal and tumoral tissue, while in other normal kidney samples chromosome patterns were normal but the corresponding tumour showed clear abnormalities (4 cases). In no cases were abnormalities found in normal kidney alone.

No correlation between the chromosome abnormality, when present, and tumour stage of evolution of the neoplastic disease could be reliably identified (Table 7.2).

DISCUSSION

Cytogenetic analyses in sporadic RCC are increasingly reported but findings are far from conclusive.

Many papers do not report the prevalence of chromosomal aberrations in the tumoral tissue from nephrectomy specimens. Chromosome abnormalities can be expected in about 60–70%, but not all cases of RCC (57%, Wolman et al 1988; 76%, Weaver et al 1988; 66% in the present series). In

Table 7.2 Follow-up of patients stratified for pathological stage of the renal carcinoma and chromosomal abnormalities

Stage	No. of patients	Chromosome abnormalities	NED	PD/CHR	DOD
I	36	8	33	3/0	0
II	8	1	8	0/0	0
III	14	6	11	3/1	0
IV	6	5	1	4/3	2

NED: no evidence of disease
PD: progressive disease
CHR: chromosomal abnormalities in progressive cases
DOD: die of disease

our cases, chromosomal abnormalities, not infrequently different from those detected in the tumoral tissue, have been found in about 48% of normal areas of kidneys bearing the RCC, as in the series reported by Wolman et al (1988). However, the significance of these data remains unclear as in other series no chromosomal abnormalities were found in normal kidney tissue (Kovacs & Frisch 1989).

In some series, rearrangements of the short arm of chromosome 3p have been found in the majority (61–94%) of cases (Zbar et al 1987, Bergerheim et al 1989, Kovacs & Frisch 1989). Weaver et al (1988) reported trisomy 7 in about 80% of cases. Moreover, in all reports a wide variety of aberrations (translocation, inversions, deletions, etc) are described, but so far a common denominator cannot be identified.

The deletion of 3p may lead to the unmasking of a recessive locus, with consequent promotion of RCC tumorigenesis (Bergerheim et al 1989); this presumes the presence of a suppressor gene (Kovacs & Frisch 1989). The 3p rearrangements appear to only be associated with the nonpapillary form of RCC, which is more aggressive as compared to the papillary form. Cases without abnormalities of chromosome 3, may be due to other undetected mutational events. However the del (3) cannot be considered a common feature in RCC, even in its nonpapillary form, as it is present in our series in only 4 of 20 (20%) of cases showing abnormalities, and in other series in about 56% (Ljungberg et al 1991).

The epidermal growth factor (EGF) gene, located on chromosome 7, is related to the invasiveness and metastatic capacity of the tumour (Collard et al 1987); thus, polysomy 7 may lead to an overexpression of this gene. The RCC growth could be attributable to this overexpression, and this abnormality could be related to higher stages and to more malignant attitude of the disease (Weaver et al 1988). In our series, trisomy 7 was not associated with a worse prognosis or higher pathological stage or grade (Table 7.3); this is in agreement with the findings of Teyssier et al (1990) and Ljungberg et al (1991).

In our experience loss of the Y chromosome in either tumours or healthy

Table 7.3 Trisomy 7

Tumour				
Stage	Grade	Diameter (cm)	Chromosomal abnormalities	Clinical follow-up
I	I	3.5	+7, +17	NED
IV*	3	4.5	+7, −Y	NED
I	2	3	+7, −Y, +2	NED
I	2	4	+7, −Y, +10, +13,	NED
II	2	10	+7, +10, −13 t, inv	
I	2	4	+7, +5, +2, +14, +16, del(3), t	NED
III	3	8.5	+7, +21, +10, del(3), 92XXXX	PD

*Micrometastases in adrenal
NED: no evidence of disease
PD: progressive disease

tissue (11 and 7 cases respectively) was frequent. This event is common in many other tumours and also in bone marrow in healthy but very elderly subjects who, however, show a normal karyotype in all other cells (Pierre et al 1972). The possible non causal role of this loss in tumour cells remains obscure.

In the present series, a high rate of failures in cytogenetic analysis occurred (about 50%); this is in contrast to the reported rates of 14–27%. Possible explanations are: prolonged ischaemia of the kidney due to the primary clamping of the renal artery during surgery; presence of necrotic tissue in the samples; insufficiently aseptic handling of the samples; insufficient tissue.

All these factors are linked to common clinical practices and may add difficulties to the interpretation of the cytogenetic findings. Therefore cytogenetic analysis, even if it gives many data of scientific interest, should not be considered fully reliable for clinical purposes at the present time.

REFERENCES

Bergerheim U, Nordenskjold M, Collins V P 1989 Deletion mapping in human renal cell carcinoma. Cancer Res 49: 1390–1396

Collard J G, Van der Poll M, Scheffer A et al 1987 Location of genes involved in invasion and metastases on human chromosome 7. Cancer Res 47: 6666–6670

Koprowski H, Herly M, Balaban G 1985 Expression of the receptor of epidermal growth factor correlates with increased dosage of chromosome 7 in malignant melanoma. Somat Cell Mol Genet 11: 297–302

Kovacs G, Frisch S 1989 Clonal chromosomal abnormalities in tumor cells from patients with sporadic renal cell carcinoma. Cancer Res 49: 651–659

Ljungberg B, Nordenson I, Roos G 1991 Cytogenetic and flow cytometry analysis in renal cell carcinoma. Eur Urol 19: 59–64

Pierre R V, Hoagland H C 1972 Age associated aneuploidy: loss of Y chromosome from human bone marrow cells with aging. Cancer 30: 889–894
Robson C J, Churchill B M, Naderson W 1969 The results of radical nephrectomy for renal cell carcinoma. J Urol 101: 239–301
Teyssier J R, Ferre D 1990 Chromosomal changes in renal cell carcinoma. No evidence for correlation with clinical stage. Cancer Genet Cytogen 45: 197–205
Weaver D J, Michalski K, Miles J 1988 Cytogenetic analysis in renal cell carcinoma: correlation with tumor aggressiveness. Cancer Res 48: 2887–2889
Wolman S R, Camuto P M, Golimbu M et al 1988 Cytogenetic analysis, flow cytometric and ultrastructural studies of twenty-nine nonfamilial human renal cell carcinoma. Cancer Res 48: 2890–2897
Zbar B, Brauch H, Talmadge C et al 1987 Loss of alleles on loci on the short arm of chromosome 3 in renal cell carcinoma. Nature 327: 721–724

8. Genes involved in oncogenesis and drug-resistance in kidney cancer

Y. Kakehi O. Ogawa O. Yoshida

INTRODUCTION

It is currently accepted that an accumulation of genetic aberrations causing activation of oncogenes and/or inactivation of tumour suppressor genes is necessary for human carcinogenesis. In human renal cell carcinomas (RCCs), previous cytogenetic studies demonstrated that the chromosomal rearrangement of the short arm of chromosome 3 (3p) occurred not only in hereditary RCC but also in sporadic RCC. These data suggest that some tumour suppressor gene(s) which are deeply associated with genesis of RCCs exist(s) on 3p. This chapter describes our studies of frequencies of the allelic loss at 3p examined by RFLP analysis in Japanese sporadic RCC patients and correlation with histopathological subtypes.

During tumorigenesis, altered transcription of several genes occurs, but many of the mRNA species in RCCs are expressed at levels comparable to those in the proximal tubular cell and characterize its biological behaviour. One such product is P-glycoprotein (PGP), a multidrug-transporter, which seems to be associated with the intrinsic anthracycline and vinca alkaloids resistance in RCC. In the present study, we examined how far PGP is involved in natural drug-resistance phenomenon of RCC in the clinical setting.

ALLELIC LOSS AT 3p IN RCCs

Incidence of the loss of heterozygosity on chromosome 3p was evaluated using 7 polymorphic probes (Table 8.1) in 35 Japanese patients with sporadic RCCs. In 30 of 35 patients examined, DNA extracted from normal kidney tissues showed constitutional heterozygosity for at least 1 of 7 loci on chromosome 3p. Of the informative 30 patients, 16 (53%) showed loss of heterozygosity on 3p (Table 8.2). The frequency was slightly lower than those previously reported from other countries. However, the loss of heterozygosity was demonstrated in over half of our Japanese cases, suggesting that the loss of heterozygosity on 3p is a non-random event in tumorigenesis of RCC (Ogawa et al 1991).

Table 8.1 Chromosome 3p loci tested for loss of heterozygosity (Reproduced from Cancer Research 1991.)

Locus symbol[a]	Probe	Enzyme	Alleles Size (kb)	Alleles Frequency	Map location
RAF1	p627	TaqI	6.8/6.3	0.74/0.26	3p25
		BglI	4.0/3.3	0.54/0.46	
THRB(erbAβ)	pBH302	HindIII	7.0/5.5	0.33/0.67	3p24.1–p22
DNF15S2	pH3H2	HindIII	2.3/2.0	0.46/0.54	3p21
D3S2	pHF12–32	MspI	2.9/1.3, 1.6	0.83/0.17	3p21
D3S4	B67	TaqI	13/12	0.14/0.86	3pter-q21
		MspI	4.8/1.6	0.16/0.84	
D3S3	pMSI–37	MspI	4.85/3.65 + 1.2	0.04/0.96	3p14
D3S32	pEFD145.1	TaqI	9.0/4.0		3p

[a] According to the Tenth International Workshop on Human Gene Mapping

CORRELATION WITH HISTOPATHOLOGICAL PHENOTYPE

Of the 30 informative patients, 16 tumours were histopathologically classified as the clear cell type. Among these, allelic loss at the 3p loci was found in 12 (75%) cases. On the other hand, allelic loss at the 3p loci was demonstrated in 1 of 7 (14%) granular cell type RCCs. This incidence was significantly lower than that in clear cell type RCCs ($p < 0.01$) (Ogawa et al 1991). All 5 patients with mixed cell type tumour were informative at RAF1 or erbA-beta locus. Of these, 3 cases containing predominantly clear cell components showed loss of heterozygosity. In contrast, the other 3 cases, consisting predominantly of granular cell components, retained heterozygosity at the 3p loci.

Table 8.2 Histopathological features and loss of heterozygosity on chromosome 3p (Reproduced from Cancer Research 1991.)

	No. of cases with loss of heterozygosity/no. of informative cases (%)
All cases	16/30 (53)
Cell type[a]	
Clear cell	12/16 (75)
Granular cell	1/7 (14)
Mixed cell	2/5 (40)
Other	1/2 (50)
Configuration[b]	
Papillary	0/3 (0)
Nonpapillary	16/27 (60)
Cytological grade	
1	11/21 (52)
2	4/7 (57)
3	1/2 (50)

[a] Clear vs. granular ($P < 0.01$)
[b] Dominant architectural configuration

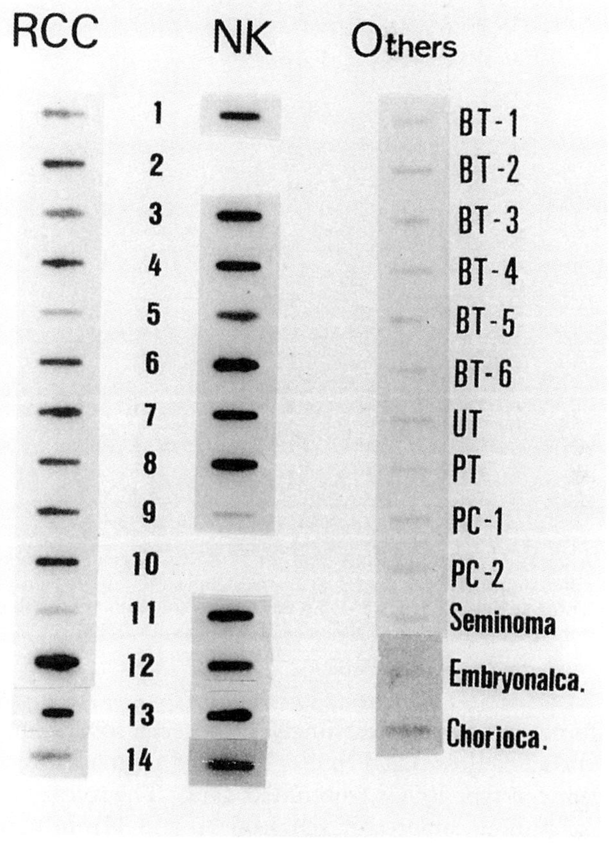

Fig. 8.1 Slot blots of 14 renal cell carcinomas (RCCs), 12 adjacent kidney tissues (NK), and 13 other urogenital tumours: BT, bladder tumour; UT, ureteral tumour; PT, renal pelvic tumour; PC, prostatic cancer. Some 10 μg of total cellular RNA were applied to each slot and hybridized with human MDR1 and cDNA fragment 5A.

As compared with nonpapillary type RCCs, papillary type RCCs infrequently showed loss of the 3p loci. However, there was no correlation of the loss of heterozygosity at 3p with either architectural configuration or cytological grading. In addition, there was no definite correlation between the tumour stages and the incidence of allelic loss at 3p.

ALLELIC LOSSES AT OTHER LOCI

We have also been studying the incidence of the allelic losses at chromosome 17p in RCC cases. Allelic losses at 17p were detected in only 6 of 36

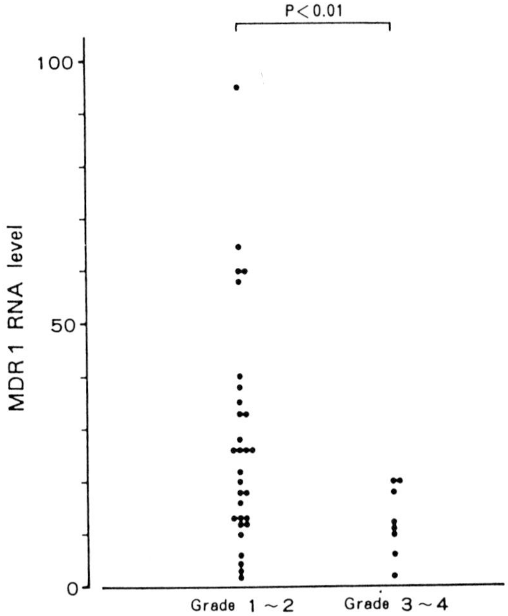

Fig. 8.2 Distribution of MDR1 RNA levels in 38 RCCs by grade of lesion. Mean level for 30 well-differentiated RCCs (grades 1–2) was significantly higher than that for 8 poorly differentiated RCCs (grades 3–4) by non-paired student's t-test. (Reproduced with permission from the Journal of the National Cancer Institute 1989.)

(17%) informative cases. Interestingly, however, a significantly higher incidence of the allelic losses at 17p was observed in granular cell type RCCs than in clear cell type RCCs (submitted data). The roles and mutual relationships of tumour suppressor genes on 3p and 17p in tumorigenesis of RCC remain to be elucidated.

MDR1 RNA LEVELS IN GENITOURINARY TUMOURS

Figure 8.1 shows slot blot analyses of RNAs extracted from genitourinary tumours using the human multidrug-resistance gene (MDR1) cDNA fragment 5A as a hybridization probe (kindly gifted by Dr I. Pastan, NIH, NCI). Only in the RCC samples, were the MDR1 RNA levels frequently elevated up to the level of the normal kidney tissue (Kakehi et al 1988, Kakehi & Yoshida 1991).

CORRELATION OF MDR1 RNA LEVELS IN RCCs WITH TUMOUR GRADES

The MDR1 RNA levels in 38 RCC samples of primary lesions were analyzed by slot blots. The arbitrary units of the MDR1 RNA level were

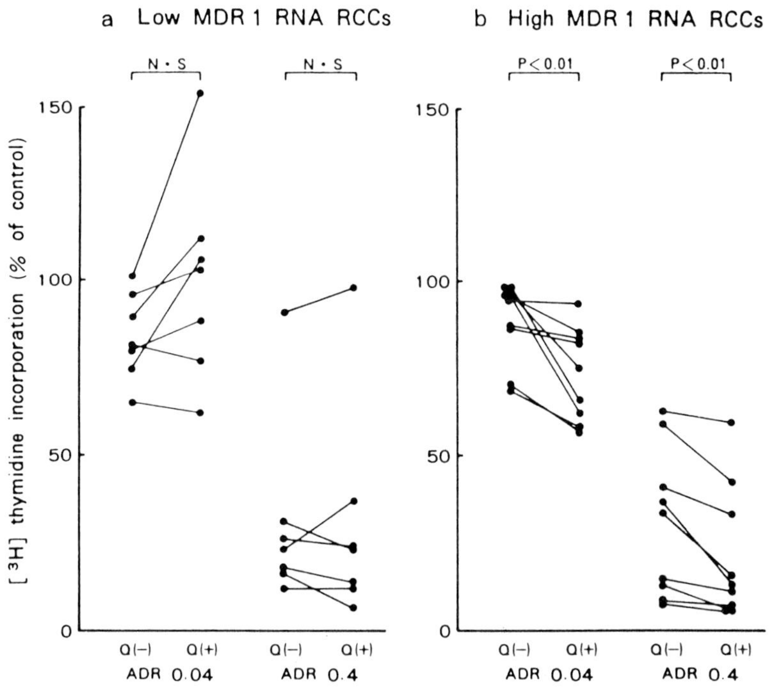

Fig. 8.3 Effect of 7.5 μg/ml quinidine (Q) on in vitro sensitivity to doxorubicin (ADR) in 16 RCC samples, which were divided into a group with low levels of MDR1 RNA or a group with high MDR1 RNA levels. (Reproduced with permission from the Journal of the National Cancer Institute 1989.)

determined by comparison with those of the multidrug-resistant KB-8-5 cells and its drug-sensitive parent, KB-3-1 cells. Figure 8.2 shows distribution of MDR1 RNA levels in 38 RCCs by grade of lesion. Mean level for 30 grade 1–2 RCCs was significantly higher than that of 8 grade 3–4 RCCs (Kanamaru et al 1989). These results are compatible with the premise that the increased expression of MDR1 gene in RCC originates from the elevated expression in renal proximal tubular cells.

REVERSING EFFECT OF QUINIDINE ON DOXORUBICIN RESISTANCE IN RCC

Some calcium-channel blockers and calmodulin antagonists, quinidine, and several other agents are known to reverse the multi-drug-resistance phenotype in vitro. We examined the enhancing effect of quinidine on sensitivity to doxorubicin in tumour explants from 16 RCC samples by scintillation assay in relation to MDR1 gene expression. The 16 RCC samples were arbitrarily divided into the high-MDR1 RNA group and the low-MDR1 RNA group. As shown in Figure 8.3, sensitivity to doxorubicin was significantly enhanced by the addition of quinidine (7.5 μg/ml) in the high-MDR1 RNA group but not in the low-MDR1 RNA group (Kanamaru et al 1989). These results suggest that PGP plays an important role in the intrinsic drug resistance of RCCs in the clinical setting.

CONCLUSION

Among genetic events during tumorigenesis of RCC, aberrations involving loci of the short arm of chromosome 3 seem to be strongly associated with clear cell type RCCs. Allelic losses at other chromosomal loci including 17p and their relation to histological phenotype remains to be clarified.

In spite of such genetic events, the MDR1 gene continues to be expressed at high levels in many RCCs and seems to be strongly associated with the intrinsic drug-resistance phenomenon.

REFERENCES

Kakehi Y, Kanamaru H, Yoshida O et al 1988 Measurement of multidrug-resistance messenger RNA in urogenital cancers; elevated expression in renal cell carcinoma is associated with intrinsic drug resistance. J Urol 139: 862–865

Kakehi Y, Yoshida O 1991 Molecular basis and clinical relevance of MDR1 gene expression in renal cell carcinoma. In: Debruyne F M J, Bukowski R M, Pontes J E et al (eds) Immunotherapy of renal cell carcinoma. Springer-Verlag, Berlin

Kanamaru H, Kakehi Y, Yoshida O et al 1989 MDR1 RNA levels in human renal cell carcinomas: correlation with grade and prediction of reversal of doxorubicin resistance by quinidine in tumor explants. J Nat Cancer Inst 81: 844–849

Ogawa O, Kakehi Y, Ogawa K 1991 Allelic loss at chromosome 3p characterizes clear cell phenotype of renal cell carcinoma. Cancer Res 51: 949–953

9. Abnormal expression of proteasomes (multicatalytic proteinase complexes) in human renal cancers

H. Kanayama K. Uema T. Inai H. Takigawa
K. Kurokawa S. Kagawa K. Tanaka A. Ichihara

INTRODUCTION

Proteasomes (multicatalytic proteinase complexes) are eukaryotic ring-shaped particles of 20S that are assumed to be responsible for the metabolism of both protein and RNAs. Recently, they were demonstrated to catalyze the degradation of abnormal and short-lived proteins such as products of the proto-oncogenes (c-myc, c-myb, c-fos), anti-oncogene (p53) and cyclin in ATP/ubiquitin-dependent fashion (Fig. 9.1). To clarify their involvement and tumorigenesis of the kidney, we examined their expression at mRNA and protein levels using cDNAs and specific antibodies against human proteasomes that have been isolated by us.

MATERIAL AND METHODS

NORTHERN BLOT ANALYSIS

Purification of RNAs

Total RNAs were extracted from normal and neoplastic parts of the tissues resected from 10 patients with renal cell carcinomas, and 6 cultured cells

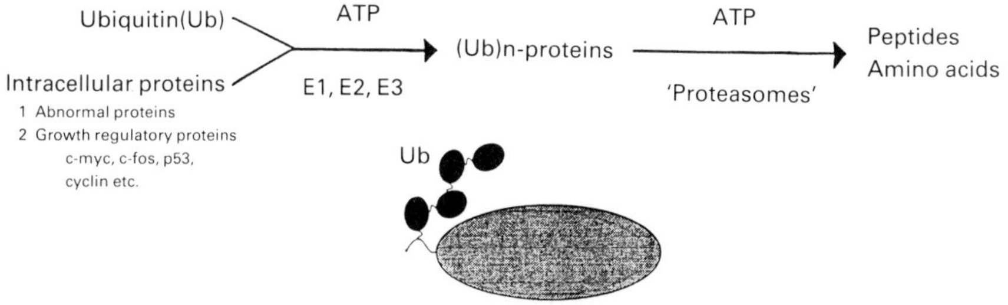

Fig. 9.1 Intracellular ATP/ubiquitin-dependent proteolytic pathway

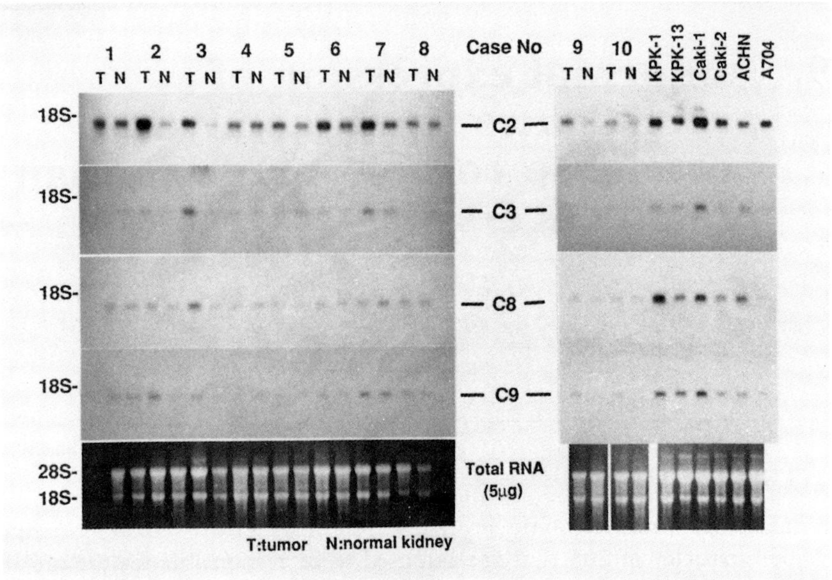

Fig. 9.2 Northern blot analysis of proteasomes in human renal cancers. Levels of mRNAs for proteasome subunits were measured by Northern blot analysis in normal (N) and neoplastic (T) parts of the kidneys of 10 patients with various renal cell carcinomas and 6 renal cancer cell lines. RNA blot hybridization and the probes used for measuring mRNAs of proteasome subunits C2, C3, C8 and C9 are described in 'Materials and Methods'. The lower panel shows the pattern of total RNA stained with ethidiun bromide. The positions of ribosomal RNAs (28S, and 18S) are indicated on the left. (Modified from Kanayama et al 1991)

established from human renal cancers by the guanidinium thiocyanate/cesium chloride method.

Electrophoresis

Samples of 5 μg of RNA were denatured and separated by electrophoresis on 1.0% agarose gel containing formaldehyde. The RNAs were then transferred to a nylon membrane.

Probes

The cDNAs cloned by us for the subunit C2, C3, C8 and C9 of rat proteasomes were used for probes.

IMMUNOLOGICAL METHODS

Samples

Normal and neoplastic parts of the kidneys of patients with primary renal cancers were homogenized in 50 mM Tris HCI buffer (pH 7.4) containing

Table 9.1 Clinical and pathological data on patients with various renal cell carcinomas and gene expressions and contents of proteasome in normal and neoplastic parts of their kidneys

Case No.	Age	Sex[a]	Histology[b]	Metastasis	Gene expression of subunit C2(T/N[c])	Proteasomes[d] (μg^e/mg protein) Tumour tissue	Normal tissue
1	72	M	Unknown	(−)	↑		
2	70	M	Clear cell, G1	(−)	↑↑↑		
3	75	F	Granular cell, G2	(−)	↑↑		
4	58	F	Clear cell, G1	(−)	→		
5	47	F	Clear cell, G1	(−)	↑	8.2	6.8
6	61	F	Clear cell, G1	(−)	↑↑	7.5	7.5
7	65	M	Granular cell, G1	(+)bone	↑↑	7.8	6.2
8	75	M	Clear cell, G1	(−)	→		
9	58	M	Clear cell, G1	(+)bone	↑↑	5.5	6.9
10	38	M	Clear cell, G1	(−)	↑	9.0	9.2
11	55	M	Mixed, G2	(+)liver		6.9	7.2
12	57	M	Clear cell, G1	(−)		3.8	6.6
13	76	M	Clear cell, G1	(−)		8.2	7.2
14	58	M	Pleomorphic, G3	(+)lung		5.6	7.7

[a] M: male, F: female
[b] Cell type and histological grade were determined according to the Japanese Pathological Society
[c] T: tumour, N: normal kidney
[d] Proteasome contents were measured quantitatively by enzyme immunoassay as described in 'Materials and Methods'
[e] μg equivalents of human liver enzyme
(Modified from Kanayama et al 1991)

1 mM dithiothreitol and 0.25 M sucrose. The homogenates were then centrifuged at 20 000 × g for 30 minutes at 4°C, and the resulting supernatants were used for examinations. Cell lysates of cultured cells were prepared by a similar procedure.

Antibodies

Human liver proteasomes were purified and injected into rabbits to generate polyclonal antisera. Monoclonal antibody against the purified human liver proteasomes was produced in mouse hybridoma cells by a standard method.

The proteasome content of the tissues and cells

The proteasome content was measured by sandwich enzyme immunoassay with monoclonal and polyclonal antibodies. Samples were prepared as above.

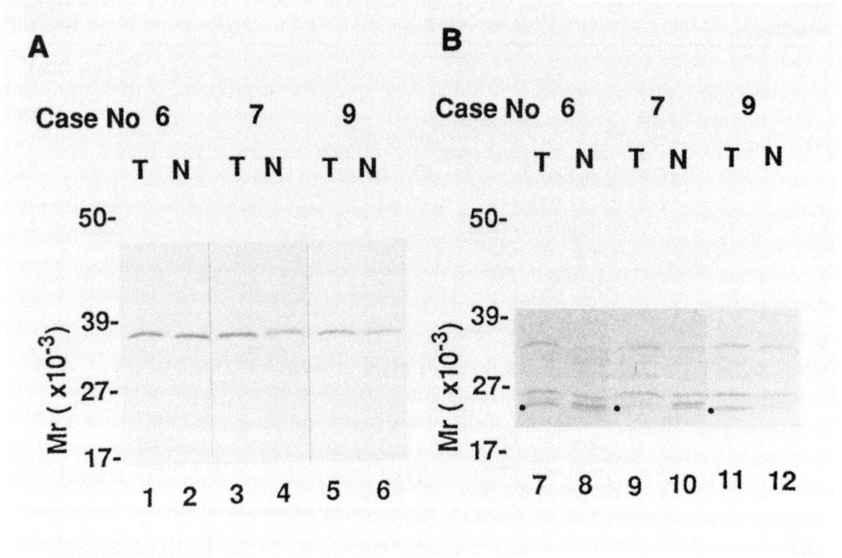

Fig. 9.3 Immunoblot analysis of proteasomes in normal(N) and neoplastic (T) parts of patients with renal cell carcinomas. Immunoblot analyses of 3 patients were performed with monoclonal antibodies to subunit C2 (lanes 1–6) and polyclonal antisera (lanes 7–12). 100 µg of soluble proteins extracted from tissues resected operatively were examined. Alteration of subunits conformation (•) of proteasomes in neoplastic parts (T) were observed with polyclonal antisera in all 3 patients examined (lanes 7, 9 and 11)

Immunoblot analysis

Samples extracted from tissues and cells were separated by SDS-PAGE in 10–20% gradient gel, and then transferred electrophoretically to Durapore membrane. The membranes were pretreated with Block Ace and then treated with monoclonal or polyclonal antibodies, and anti-mouse or anti-rabbit IgGs conjugated with alkaline phosphatase. They were then stained by the alkaline phosphatase reaction.

Immunoprecipitations

Cultured cells were labelled by ^{35}S-methionine for 3 hours in CO_2 incubator and cell extracts were precipitated by monoclonal antibody. Then, the resulting precipitates were subjected to SDS-PAGE (10–20% gradient gel), and after electrophoresis the gel was dried and subjected to fluorography.

Immunohistochemical and immunocytochemical staining

Tissues obtained surgically from patients were fixed with 10% neutralized formaldehyde in 0.1 M phosphate buffer and embedded in paraffin. Serial sections of tissues were treated with mixtures of four monoclonal antibodies

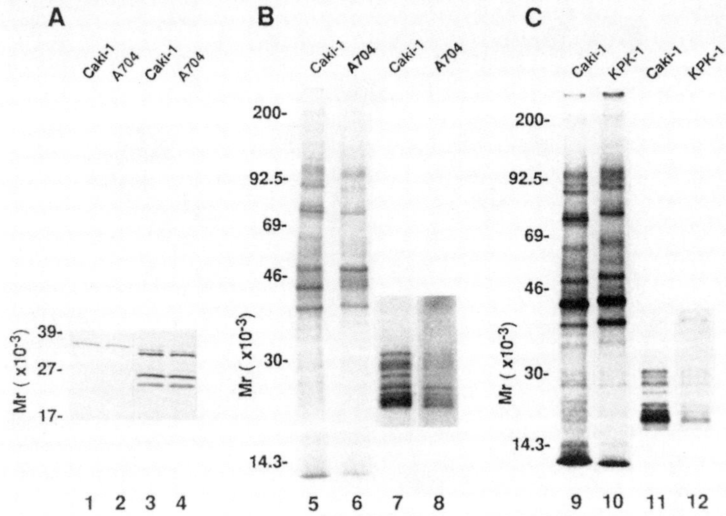

Fig. 9.4 Immunoblot analyses and immunoprecipitations of proteasomes in renal cancer cell lines. **A** Immunoblot analyses of Caki-1 and A704 cells with monoclonal (lanes 1 and 2) and polyclonal (lanes 3 and 4) antibodies. The cell extracts (100 μg) were used for immunoelectrophoretic-blot analyses. **B** and **C** [^{35}S]-methionine incorporation into proteasomes of Caki-1 (lanes 7 and 11), A704 (lane 8) and KPK-1 (lane 12). Samples of the 3 cell extracts with the same radioactivity (5×10^6 cpm) were used for immunoprecipitation analysis to measure proteasome synthesis. Increased proteasome synthesis correlated to gene expressions of subunit C2 were observed in Caki-1 cells (lanes 7 and 11). (Modified from Kanayama et al 1990)

against human proteasomes, and proteasomes were detected by the avidin-biotin-peroxidase complex (ABC) method. Cultured cells were fixed with cold methanol and proteasomes were stained by the same method.

RESULTS AND CONCLUSIONS

Enhanced gene expression of proteasomes were observed in 8 neoplastic parts resected from 10 patients with renal cell carcinomas, and in all 6 cultured cells examined (Fig. 9.2). However, no significant difference was found by enzyme immunoassay in the proteasomal contents of cancerous and normal parts of kidney (Table 9.1). But immuno-electrophoretic blot analysis showed that the subunit composition of proteasomes was altered in kidney tumours as compared with those of normal parts (Fig. 9.3).

It was suggested from the results of immunoblot analysis and immunoprecipitations in 3 different cell lines that the levels of MRNAs for the subunits of proteasomes were correlated with the activities of proteasome synthesis (Fig. 9.4).

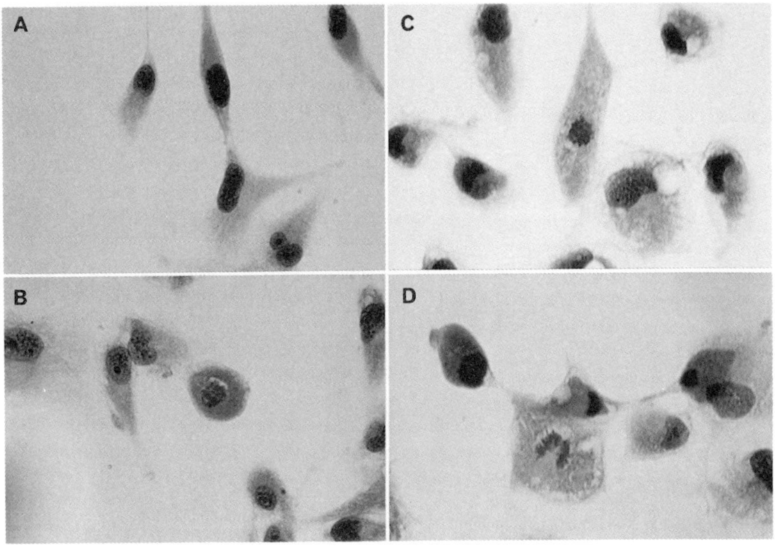

Fig. 9.5 Immunocytochemical staining of proteasomes in human renal cancer cell lines (×400). Caki-1 (**A** and **B**) and A704 (**C** and **D**) cells were fixed with methanol and treated with mixtures of 4 monoclonal antibodies against human proteasomes. Then, cells were stained by ABC methods and counter-stained with Mayer's haematoxylin. High concentrations of proteasomes in the nuclei and their diffuse distributions in the cytoplasm of Caki-1 and A704 cells were observed.

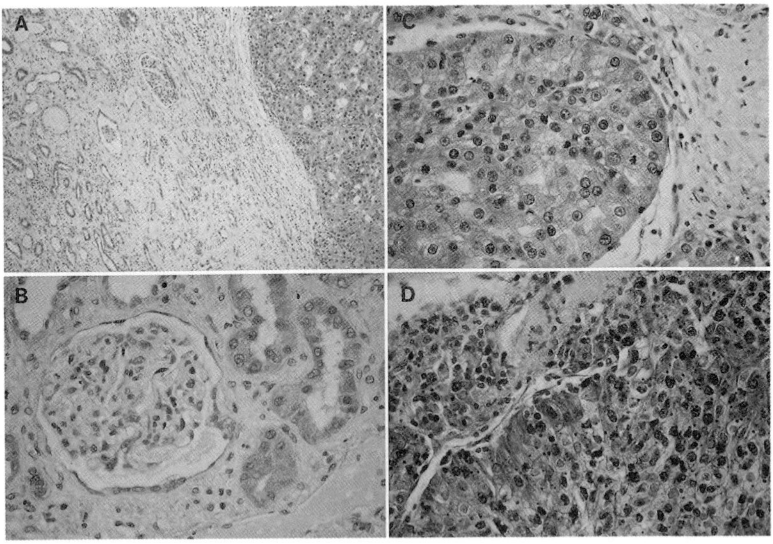

Immunohistochemical and immunocytochemical staining with anti-proteasome monoclonal antibody showed considerably increased concentrations of proteasomes in tumour cells, in which proteasomes were found mostly in the nuclei (Figs 9.5 and 9.6).

These results suggest that the proteasome-mediated system is functionally involved in the cancerous state in human kidney.

REFERENCE

Kanayama H et al 1991 Changes in expressions of proteasome and ubiquitin in human renal cancer cells. Cancer Res 51: 6680.

Fig. 9.6 (see facing page) Immunohistochemical staining of proteasomes in human renal cell carcinomas (**A** × 100, **B**, **C** and **D** × 400). Tissues obtained surgically from patients (A, B and C: case no. 11, D: case no. 2) were fixed with 10% neutralized formaldehyde and embedded in paraffin. Serial sections of the tissues were treated with mixtures of culture media containing 4 monoclonal antibodies against human proteasomes and then stained by avidin-biotin-peroxidase complex (ABC) method. After enzyme staining, specimens were counter-stained with Mayer's hematoxylin. Immunohistochemical staining of specimens of normal parts of the kidney (A and B) showed that proteasomes are present at considerably high levels in cells of renal tubules and epithelial cells of the collecting duct, but not in the gromerulus. And abnormally high levels of proteasomes were found in cancerous parts of renal cell carcinomas (C and D).

10. Bladder cancer survival and human papillomavirus infection. Immunohistochemistry and in-situ hybridization

A. Lopez-Beltran J. C. Carrasco-Aznar
C. Reymundo C. Morales-Jimenez M. Toro-Rojas
R. Lopez-Pardo M. Santamaria Ossorio

SUMMARY

The aim of the present research was to investigate human papillomavirus infection by means of immunohistochemistry and in-situ hybridization in 76 bladder cancer specimens, and to correlate results with clinical parameters, such as patients' survival and tumour recurrences. A biotinylated DNA probe that recognizes HPV 6–11, HPA 16–18, and HPV 31–33–35 was used for in-situ hybridization. A polyclonal antibody recognizing human papillomavirus structural antigen was used for immunohistochemistry. In-situ hybridization and immunohistochemistry were developed by alkaline phosphatase and immunogold-silver techniques, respectively. Our results showed that 26 (34.2%) out of 76 bladder carcinoma specimens reacted with human papillomavirus structural antigen by immunohistochemistry, which significantly correlated with patients' survival ($p = 0.005$) and tumour recurrences ($p = 0.046$). In-situ hybridization data were available in 18 out of 26 cases that had previously reacted with human papillomavirus structural antigen. Nine (50%) out of 18 such cases were positive for human papillomavirus types 16–18, which significantly correlated also with patients' survival ($p = 0.025$) and tumour recurrences ($p = 0.020$). No positive signals were found for HPV types 6–11 or 31–33–35 DNA probes.

These observations may prove useful in prognostic stratification of patients with bladder cancer.

INTRODUCTION

Recent advances in molecular biology have enabled researchers to identify a specific type of human papillomavirus (HPV) genome or its expression within HPV-associated lesions (Mevorach et al 1990). Currently, 60 types of HPV have been identified (Chang 1990), with types 6, 11, 16, 18 and 31 accounting for 80–90% of the clinically manifest genitourinary lesions (Mevorach et al 1990). Transitional cell carcinoma of the urinary bladder is common, although its aetiology is not completely understood (Bryant et al 1987, Lopez-Beltran et al 1989, 1991). The bladder is particularly vulnerable to environmental carcinogens, and many factors have been identified as probable causes of bladder cancer (Hoover & Strasser 1980, Morrison 1984, Gonzalez et al 1985). While viral studies on mammalian urothelium have shown an association between the bovine papillomavirus and cancer of the bladder in cattle (Olson et al 1965), the evidence for HPV involvement in urinary bladder cancer in man is less clear (Bryant et al 1991). The presence of HPV structural antigen in cancer of the bladder has previously been established (Bryant et al 1987). However, although HPV DNA types 6 and 11 have been identified in condylomata acuminata and cancers of the bladder and urethra (Del Mistro et al 1988, Querci della Rovere el al 1988, Mevorachet al 1990, Wilson et al 1990), and the presence of HPV types 16 and 18 in urinary bladder carcinomas has been established (Kitamura et al 1988, Bryant et al 1991), the prognostic significance of such findings has yet to be substantiated.

The aim of the present research was to investigate human papillomavirus infection in 76 bladder cancer specimens by means of immunohistochemistry (detecting HPV structural antigen), and in-situ hybridization histochemistry (using a biotinylated DNA probe specific for HPV types 6 and 11, HPV types 16 and 18, and HPV types 31, 33 and 35), and then to correlate results with prognostic parameters, such as patients' survival and tumour recurrences.

MATERIAL AND METHODS

The study included a group of 76 unselected and consecutive cases of transitional cell carcinoma of the urinary bladder from the files of Cordoba General Hospital. All the 76 patients underwent transurethral resection. Their mean age was 66.57 $\pm$ 1.17. Fourteen patients were female. Selected tissue specimens from all biopsies, formalin-fixed paraffin embedded, were analyzed for pathological grade and stage. All cases were followed for at least five years.

Immunohistochemical expression of HPV structural antigen was determined by a modification of the immunogold-silver staining method (Holgate et al 1983). Briefly, after de-waxing with xylene and hydration with grading alcohols through distilled water, the reactions were washed in PBS, treated with normal goat serum in a 1/200 dilution for 20 minutes, and then incubated overnight (18 h) at 4°C with primary antibody (rabbit anti-HPV, Biogenex Laboratories, San Ramon, CA, USA) in a 1/100 dilution. The treatment with the first antibody was followed by the secondary biotinylated antibody (goat anti-rabbit IgG, Janssen Biotech NV, B–2430 Olen, Belgium), and then the Auroprobe-LM-streptavidin (Janssen Biotech NV, B–2430 Olen, Belgium). The deposited gold particles were enlarged using the Intense-M-Silver-enhancement kit (Janssen Biotech NV, B–2430 Olen, Belgium). Silver precipitation was observed under the microscope within 15 minutes, and the reaction stopped by immersion in distilled water. The sections were counterstained with eosine. A case of genitourinary condylomata acuminata was used as positive control. The replacement of the primary antibody by the immunoglobulin fraction on nonimmunized rabbit serum in a 1/100 dilution (Dakopatt, Denmark) was used as negative control.

In-situ hybridization was carried out using Vira-Type-HPV tissue-hybridization kit and Vira-Type-HPV DNA probes (Life Technologies Inc, Gaithersburg, MD 20877 USA). The Vira-Type-HPV-tissue-hybridization system uses a streptavidin-alkaline-phosphatase conjugate in which the chromagen is 5–bromo–4-chloro–3-indolylphosphate in the presence of nitroblue tetrazolium. The Vira-Type-HPV DNA probe is a biotin-based probe detecting HPV types 6–11. HPA types 16–18, and HPV types 31–33–35. The posthybridization wash and hybridization is done under low stringency. The conditions recommended by the manufacturer for hybridization and detection were strictly followed. Briefly, serial sections were placed on slides pretreated with 2% solution of organosilane in acetone (Nuovo & Richart 1989). The tissue sections were deparaffinized, hydrated, air dried, and then treated with the proteinase solution (2 mg/ml) included in the tissue hybridization kit. After denaturing the respective HPV DNA probes cocktail and tissue together at 100°C for 8 minutes, the hybridization reaction went for two hours at 37°C beneath glass coverslips. The coverslips were removed, sections washed at 37°C in two changes of buffer saline solution containing bovine serum albumin at 37°C, followed by signal detection as recommended. Then, the sections were counterstained with eosine, dehydrated in absolute alcohol, cleared in xylene, and mounted in permanent medium. A positive DNA control probe specific for human genomic DNA sequences was used in each tissue biopsy. The positive DNA control probe allows evaluation of tissue fixation, digestion and denaturation, all of which affect the availability of target DNA. Furthermore, a case of genitourinary condylomata acuminata reactive with HPV DNA types 16–11 was used as positive control. A negative DNA control probe was also included in the present study to aid in the interpretation of weak signals.

The bivariate statistical analysis was undertaken using Chi-square and Fisher tests.

RESULTS

The selected variables representative of the 76 transitional cell carcinomas included in this study are illustrated in Tables 10.1, 10.2 and 10.3. Immunohistochemical staining of bladder tumour sections with HPV

Table 10.1 Frequency distribution of selected variables under study according to patients' survival status

Factors	Categories	No. deceased (%)	No. alive (%)	p-value	No. overall (%)
Patients		19(100.0)	57(100.0)		76(100.0)
Age*	M ± SD†	66.84 ± 2.45	66.48 ± 1.34		66.57 ± 1.17
Sex	Male	15(79.0)	47(82.5)		62(81.6)
	Female	4(21.0)	10(17.5)		14(18.4)
Grade	Low	4(21.0)	38(66.7)		42(55.3)
	High	15(79.0)	19(33.3)		34(44.7)
	Low vs high			0.001	
Stage	Low	7(38.9)	45(78.9)		52(69.3)
	High	11(61.1)	12(21.1)		23(30.7)
	Low vs high			0.004	
HPV pAb	+ve	12(63.2)	14(24.6)		26(34.2)
	−ve	7(36.8)	43(75.4)		50(65.8)
	+ve vs −ve			0.005	

* Age at diagnosis (years). † Mean ± Standard Deviation

structural antigen using an immunogold-silver staining technique produced black nuclear staining in 26 (34.2%) of the samples studied (Table 10.1), which significantly correlated with patients' survival status ($p = 0.005$). A significant statistical relationship was also found ($p = 0.046$) to a positive HPV structural antigen immunoreactivity in recurrent tumours of the urinary bladder (Table 10.2). In-situ hybridization data were available in 18 out of 26 cases that had previously reacted with HPV structural antigen. No signal was detected using the HPV type 6–11 or 31–33–35 DNA probes. However, positive hybridization signals were detected in 9 (50%) out of 18 such investigated cases when the sections were hybridized with the HPV type 16–18 DNA probe, which significantly correlated with

Table 10.2 Frequency distribution of selected variables according to tumour recurrences

Factors	Categories	Recurrence No. (%)	No recurrence No. (%)	p-value	Overall No. (%)
Patients		31(100.0)	36(100.0)		67(100.0)
Age*	M ± SD†	70.27 ± 1.64	63.69 ± 1.60		66.68 ± 1.21
Sex	Male	25(80.6)	29(80.6)		54(80.6)
	Female	6(19.4)	7(19.4)		13(19.4)
	Male vs female			0.764	
Grade	Low	13(41.9)	28(77.8)		41(61.2)
	High	18(58.1)	8(22.2)		26(38.8)
	Low vs high			0.006	
Stage	Low	21(67.7)	31(86.1)		52(77.6)
	High	10(32.3)	5(13.9)		15(22.4)
	Low vs high			0.132	
HPV pAb	+ve	16(51.6)	9(25.0)		25(37.3)
	−ve	15(48.4)	27(75.0)		42(62.7)
	+ve vs −ve			0.046	

* Age at diagnosis (years) †Mean ± Standard Deviation

Table 10.3 Frequency distribution of selected variables according to HPV DNA types 16–18 investigated by in-situ hybridization (ISH) histochemistry

Factors	Categories	ISH +ve No. (%)	ISH −ve No. (%)	p-value	Overall No. (%)
Patients		9(100.0)	9(100.0)		18(100.0)
Age*	M ± SD†	64.56 ± 4.69	61.33 ± 3.65		62.94 ± 2.91
Sex	Male	7(77.8)	8(88.9)		15(83.3)
	Female	2(22.2)	1(11.1)		3(16.7)
	Male vs female			0.500	
Grade	Low	2(22.2)	5(55.6)		7(38.9)
	High	7(77.8)	4(44.4)		11(61.1)
	Low vs high			0.167	
Stage	Low	3(33.3)	8(99.9)		11(61.1)
	High	6(66.7)	1(11.1)		7(38.9)
	Low vs high			0.025	
Recurrence	Yes	7(87.5)	2(25.0)		9(56.3)
	No	1(12.5)	6(75.0)		7(43.7)
	Yes vs no			0.020	
Survival	Deceased	6(66.7)	1(11.1)		7(38.9)
	Alive	3(33.3)	8(88.9)		11(61.1)
	Deceased vs alive			0.025	

* Age at diagnosis (years) †Mean ± Standard Deviation

patients' survival ($p = 0.025$) and tumour recurrences ($p = 0.020$) (Table 10.3). Hybridization using the negative DNA control probe was negative. Meanwhile, hybridization of the positive DNA control probe was positive, as well as the additional positive control condylomata acuminata which reacted with HPV types 6–11 DNA probe.

DISCUSSION

Bladder cancer is considered a result of environmental carcinogens, some of which may increase bladder cancer risk 10–50 fold (Shulte et al 1985, Hoover & Strasser 1980, Gonzalez et al 1985). Cancer of the urinary bladder is one of the commonest malignancies in occidental males (Bryant et al 1991). Epidemiological, pathological and clinical evidence supports the pathogenesis of bladder cancer as a multi-stage process, with an often unpredictable course (Lopez-Beltran et al 1989, 1991), characterized by a significant number of recurrences and frequent evolution towards infiltrating disease (Abel 1988). The association of HPV with premalignant lesions has long been recognized, and such lesions are found throughout the genitourinary tract (Syrjanen 1990). Human papillomaviruses are known to infect man, and although most of these proliferations are benign, some may convert to malignancies; this conversion is related to HPV type. In the genitourinary tract, HPV types 6–11 are most commonly associated with genital condylomata acuminata, whereas types 16–18 are associated with dysplasias and carcinomas (Chang 1990).

Human papillomavirus structural antigen has been detected in 16–50% of cases of cervical intra-epithelial neoplasia (Singer et al 1985). However, recent work has shown that 96% of such tumours contain HPV DNA, when appropriate DNA in-situ hybridization techniques are applied (Kadish et al 1986). Therefore immunohistochemical detection of HPV structural antigen may not provide the best estimate of the extent of involvement of human HPV in bladder neoplasia (Bryant et al 1987). The last instance may be corroborated by our results, even though the immunogold-silver staining method is very sensitive (Holgate et al 1983). Crossreactivity with non-specific antigens is a common finding when polyclonal antibodies are used for immunohistochemistry. This, and other related studies used rabbit polyclonal antibodies (Bryant et al 1987, Murphy et al 1983) which may explain the low sensitivity found by Bryant et al (1987), corroborated our results. These differences are notable when immunohistochemical data care compared with HPV DNA in-situ hybridization histochemistry for specific HPV types 6–11 and 16–18 (Bryant et al 1991). Our results also corroborate previous reports on HPV types present in the urothelium. HPV DNA types 6–11 have previously been identified in condylomata acuminata and occasionally in cancers of the bladder and urethra (Del Mistro et al 1988, Querci della Rovere et al 1988, Mevorach et al 1990, Wilson et al 1990). Our study failed to demonstrate bladder tumours positive for HPV DNA types 6–11, thus supporting the concept that HPV types 6–11 are closely associated with benign lesions, with only a few examples of HPV types 6–11 illustrated in transitional cell carcinomas of the urinary bladder (Del Mistro et al 1988, Querci della Rovere et al 1988, Mevorach et al 1990, Bryant et al 1991). In contrast, HPV DNA types 16–18 were identified in a number of transitional cell carcinomas of the bladder corroborating previous research (Kitamura et al 1988, Bryant et al 1991). We also failed to identify transitional cell carcinomas reactive with HPV DNA types 31–33–35. Our research was intended to correlate the results on HPV expression by immunohistochemistry and DNA in-situ hybridization with major prognostic parameters including patients' survival and tumour recurrences. However, although we found that both the HPV structural antigen immunoreactivity and the HPV DNA types 16–18 expression correlated significantly with poor survival and high tumour recurrences, we failed to demonstrate any significant relationship with the pathological grade and stage. This suggests that the expression of human papillomavirus by transitional cell carcinomas of the urinary bladder may represent an important prognostic parameter, which seems to be independent of the morphological prognostic factors represented by pathological grade and stage. However, although this study has shown the presence of human papillomavirus in transitional cell carcinomas of the bladder, further studies will be necessary in order more fully to assess the role that these and other HPV types may have in the genesis of these tumours. Furthermore, the possibility of investigating the presence of HPV DNA by more sensitive molecular techniques such as a polymerase chain reaction, makes the determination of the presence of HPV sequences in these tumours of great interest. Such studies are now in progress.

ACKNOWLEDGEMENT

This research was supported in part by the grants 02–90–07, Hospital Reina Sofia, Cordoba, Spain, and DGICYT-SM89-0011.

We thank Pilar Camo for his excellent technical assistance.

REFERENCES

Abel P O 1988 Prognostic indices in transitional cell carcinoma of the bladder. A review. Br J Urol 62: 103–109

Bryant P, Davies P, Wilson D 1991 Detection of human papillomavirus DNA in cancer of the urinary bladder by in-situ hybridisation. Br J Urol 68: 49–52

Bryant P, Skelly J, Wilson D 1987 Demonstration of papillomavirus structural antigen in human urinary bladder neoplasia. Br Urol 60: 405–409

Chang F 1990 Role of papillomaviruses. J Clin Pathol 43: 269–276

Del Mistro A, Koss L G, Braunstein J et al 1988 Condylomata acuminata of the urinary bladder. Natural history, viral typing and DNA content. Am J Surg Pathol 12: 205–215

Gonzalez C, Lopez-Abente G, Errezola M et al 1985 Occupation, tobacco use, coffee, and bladder cancer in the county Mataró (Spain). Cancer 55: 2031–2034

Holgate C S, Jackson P, Cowen P et al 1983 Immunogold-silver staining: new method of immunostaining with enhanced sensitivity. J Histochem Cytochem 31: 938–944

Hoover R N, Strasser P H 1980 Artificial sweeteners and human bladder cancer. Lancet I: 837–840

Kadish A S, Burk R D, Kress Y et al 1986 Human papillomaviruses of different types in precancerous lesions of the uterine cervix. Hum Pathol 17: 384–392

Kitamura T, Yogo Y, Ueki T et al 1988 Presence of human papillomavirus type 16 genome in bladder carcinoma in situ of a patient with mild immunodeficiency. Cancer Res 48: 7207–7211

Lopez-Beltran A, Morales C, Reymundo et al 1989 T-zone histiocytes and recurrence of papillary urothelial bladder carcinoma. Urol Int 44: 205–209

Lopez-Beltran A, Croghan G A, Croghan I et al 1991 Prognostic factors in bladder cancer survival. Cancer (in press)

Mevorach R A, Cos L R, di Sant'Agnese P A et al 1990 Human papillomavirus type 6 in grade I transitional cell carcinoma of the urethra. Journal of Urology 143: 126–128

Morrison A S 1984 Advances in the aetiology of urothelial cancer. Urol Clin North 11: 557–566

Murphy W M. 1983 Current topics in the pathology of bladder cancer. Pathol Annu 18(1): 1–25

Nuovo G J, Richart R M 1989 A comparison of biotin- and ^{35}S-based in-situ hybridization methodologies for detection of human papillomavirus DNA. Lab Invest 61: 471–476

Olson C, Pamucku A M, Brobst D F 1965 Papilloma-like virus from bovine urinary bladder tumours. Cancer Res 25: 840–847

Querci della Rovere G, Oliver R T D, McCance D J et al 1988 Development of bladder tumour containing HPV type 11 DNA after renal transplantation. Br J Urol 62: 36–38

Shulte P A, Ringer K, Hemstreet G P et al 1985 Risk assessment of a cohort exposed to aromatic amines. J Occup Med 27: 115–121

Singer A, Wilters J, Walker P et al 1985 Comparison of prevalence of human papillomavirus antigen in biopsies from women with cervical intraepithelial neoplasia. J Clin Pathol 38: 855–857

Syrjanen S M 1990 Basic concepts and practical applications of recombinant DNA techniques in detection of human papillomavirus infection. APMIS 98: 95–110

Wilson R W, Chenggis M L, Under E R 1990 Longitudinal study of human papillomavirus infection of the female urogenital tract by in situ hybridization. Arch Pathol Lab Med 114: 155–159

11. The role of ras p21 oncoprotein in human bladder cancer

D. Delakas N. J. Agnantis J. Parliaras A. Cranidis D. A. Spandidos

INTRODUCTION

Abnormal expression of cellular oncogenes and onco-suppressor genes has been implicated in the development of cancer (Spandidos & Anderson 1989). The members of the ras oncogene family, Ha-, Ki- and N-ras, seem to play an important role in several human common cancers since these genes have frequently been found to be activated by qualitative or quantitative changes (Field & Spandidos 1990, Spandidos 1989). Thus, molecular hybridization analyses (Spandidos & Kerr 1984, Spandidos & Agnantis 1984, Spandidos et al 1985) and immunohistochemical studies (Agnantis et al 1986, 1988, 1991, Williams et al 1985, Viola et al 1985, 1986) have demonstrated elevated ras mRNA and ras 21 protein in tumours as compared to normal adjacent tissue. Moreover, cloned human ras genes can trigger many of the cancer cell phenotypes, i.e. cell immortalization, morphological transformation or tumorigenic conversion of recipient cells in culture (Spandidos & Wilkie 1984).

In a previous study, we examined immunohistochemically ras p21 expression in normal, hyperplastic and dysplastic bladder lesions, as well as in papillomas and transitional carcinomas. Our results showed that the dysplastic and cancerous lesions were strongly positive while the rest of the normal and benign material was negative or weakly positive (Agnantis et al 1990). In the present study we examined the relation of the ras p21 oncoprotein expression with the degree of tumour grading in bladder carcinomas. Our results suggest that p21 plays an important role in the initial stages of bladder carcinogenesis.

PATIENTS AND METHODS

Tissue sections from a total of 34 bladder carcinoma patients were examined. The tumour grading, which also expresses the degree of differentiation, was performed according to Mostofi's WHO classification.

Immunohistochemical analysis of the ras p21 protein was undertaken using the ras p21 rat monoclonal antibody (Further et al 1982). Tissue sections 5 µm thick were mounted on slides and deparaffinized. Endogenous peroxidase activity was blocked by immersing the sections for 30 min in an aqueous solution of 3% H_2O_2, and the sections were washed with PBS and treated for 10 min with human serum-PBS (1:9) at room temperature. Then the sections were treated with the Y13-259 rat monoclonal antibody diluted in human serum-PBS (1:9) (at dilution 1:50, 1:100 or 1:200 depending on the stock) for one hour at 37°C, washed twice for 5 min each and treated with streptavidin-peroxidase diluted in PBS (at a dilution 1:200) for 15 min at 37°C.

For localization of the primary antibody, 1 µg/ml of 3,3′-diaminobenzidine tetrahydrochloride solution was used. The sections were developed for 10 min at room temperature and then counterstained with Harris Haematoxilin.

As controls for the immunostaining the following two cell lines were used. CHL is the parental non-transformed Chinese hamster lung fibroblast cell line which expresses barely detectable levels of the endogenous ras p21. FH06T1–1 cells were derived from CHL cells after transfection with a recombinant plasmid pH06T1 which carries the T24 human Harvey-ras 1 gene (Spandidos & Wilkie 1984). These cells express the ras p21 at elevated levels.

RESULTS

Tissue sections from 34 bladder carcinomas were examined employing immunohistochemistry for detection of the expression of the ras p21 protein. The level of ras p21 was analyzed using the monoclonal antibody Y13-259 and the biotin-streptavidin-peroxidase-DAB technique. The intensity of staining was graded as negative or equivocal (–/+), moderate (+) or intense (+ +). A summary of the data obtained is shown in Table 11.1. Out of the 34 specimens evaluated the results can be summarized as follows:

1. All malignant lesions of stage I (2/2), I-II (11/11), II (8/8) and II-III (5/5) showed elevated expression of ras p21.
2. One out of 6 malignant lesions of stage III, and 2 out of 2 of stage IV were negative.

Table 11.1 Immunohistochemical staining of ras p21 in 34 human bladder carcinomas.

	Staining intensity (No. of cases)		
Tumour grade	–/+	+	+ +
I	–	–	2
I–II	–	4	7
II	–	1	7
II–III	–	1	4
III	1	3	2
IV	2	–	–

The ability of the Y13–259 monoclonal antibody to detect elevated levels of ras p21 was confirmed by including in all experiments the negative (CHL) and positive (FH06T1-1) cell lines as controls (see Patients and Methods).

DISCUSSION

Elevated expression of cellular ras genes has been demonstrated in a variety of human tumours using molecular hybridization (Spandidos & Kerr 1984, Spandidos & Agnantis 1984, Spandidos et al 1985) and immunohistochemical analysis (Agnantis et al 1986, 1988, 1991, Williams et al 1985, Viola et al 1985, 1986). In-vitro studies have also suggested that elevated expression of ras genes is important in cell transformation (Spandidos & Wilkie 1984).

We have previously examined, using an immunohistochemical technique, ras p21 expression in human bladder endoscopy specimens (Agnantis et al 1990). The normal urothelium tended to be negative, while the umbrella cells from the superficial layer always expressed a higher degree of positivity. The majority of the hyperplastic lesions and the papillomas were weakly positive or negative. In contrast, all the dysplastic lesions and the carcinomas were strongly positive. In the present study we examined the level of ras p21 in 34 human bladder carcinomas. Our results suggest that ras p21 oncoprotein expression is inversely related to tumour differentiation and grading, i.e. as the grading increases ras p21 expression decreases. Although, our sample is relatively small, it is tempting to suggest that the ras p21 oncoprotein is not expressed in highly malignant and/or anaplastic tumours which are composed mainly of an undifferentiated cell population. However, it does seem to play a role in the initial stages of bladder carcinogenesis.

REFERENCES

Agnantis N J, Petraki C, Markoulatos et al 1986 Immunohistochemical study of the *ras* oncogene expression in human breast lesions. Anticancer Res 6: 1157–1160

Agnantis N J, Spandidos D A, Mahera H et al 1988 Immunohistochemical study of *ras* oncogene expression in endometrial and cervical human lesions. Eur J Gynaecol Oncol 9:360–365

Agnantis N J, Konstandinidou A, Poulios C 1990 Immunohistochemical study of the *ras* oncogene expression in human bladder endoscopy specimens. Eur J Surg Oncol 16: 153–160

Agnantis N J, Apostolakis N, Sficas C 1991 Immunohistochemical detection of *ras* p21 and *myc* p62 in colonic adenomas and carcinomas. Hepato-Gastroenterology 38: 239–242

Field J K, Spandidos D A 1990. The role of *ras* and *myc* oncogenes in human solid tumours and their relevance in diagnosis and prognosis. Anticancer Res 10: 1–22

Furth M E, Davis L J, Fleurdelys B et al 1982. Monoclonal antibodies to the p21 products of the transforming gene of Harvey murine sarcoma virus of the cellular *ras* gene family. J Virol 43: 294–304

Spandidos D A, Wilkie N M 1984 Malignant transformation of early passage rodent cells by a single mutated human oncogene. Nature 310: 469–475

Spandidos D A, Kerr I B, 1984 Elevated expression of the human *ras* oncogene family in premalignant and malignant tumors of the colorectum. Br J Cancer 49: 681–688

Spandidos D A, Agnantis N J 1984 Human malignant tumors of the breast as compared to their respective normal tissue have elevated expression of the Harvey *ras* oncogene. Anticancer Res 4: 269–272

Spandidos D A 1985 Mechanism of carcinogenesis: the role of oncogenes, transcriptional enhancers and growth factors. Anticancer Res 5: 485–498

Spandidos D A 1989. *Ras* oncogenes. Plenum Press, New York. pp1–323

Spandidos D A, Anderson M L M 1989 Oncogenes and onco-suppressor genes: their involvement in cancer. J Pathol 157: 1–10

Viola M V, Fromowitz F, Oravez S et al 1985 *Ras* oncogene p21 expression is increased in premalignant lesions and high grade bladder carcinomas. J Exp Med 161: 1213–1218

Viola M V, Fromowitz F, Oravez S 1986 Expression of *ras* oncogene p21 in prostate cancer. N Engl J Med 314: 133–137

Williams A R W, Piris J, Spandidos D A et al 1985 Immunohistochemical detection of the *ras* oncogene p21 product in an experimental tumor and in human colorectal neoplasms. Br J Cancer 50: 687–693

12. Study of ras gene alterations in human bladder tumours

F. Descotes H. Bittard A. Remy-Martin
E. Khenifar M. Bittard G. L. Adessi

INTRODUCTION

Members of the ras gene family (Ha-, Ki- and N-ras) are frequently activated in many different human cancers (Nishimura et al 1987). Two possible mechanisms for ras gene activation have been described. The first is a qualitative activation by a single point mutation in codon 12 or 13 or 61 of the ras genes. These mutations cause an amino acid substitution in the ras gene product, p21 protein (Bos 1989). The second mechanism is a quantitative alteration by an increase in the copy number of the normal ras gene (Pulciani et al 1985).

The c-Ha-ras-1 gene presents a restriction fragment length polymorphism (RFLP) due to the variable tandem repetition (VTR) sequence in the 3′-flanking region (Capon et al 1983). Krontiris et al (1985) described four common allelic restriction fragments of c-Ha-ras-1 locus gene plus some rare alleles both in the white blood cell (WBC) DNA and in the tumour DNA from patients with various types of cancer. These authors demonstrated several allele distributions varying according to the cancer type, and which differed from those of a cancer-free population, with significantly more rare alleles in the cancer patients than in the cancer-free population. These results suggested that c-Ha-ras–1 RFLP may be useful to evaluate the risk of cancer. Furthermore, Fearon et al (1985) found losses of genes on the short arm of chromosome 11 and suggested the potential involvement of chromosome 11p in transitional cell carcinoma of bladder.

To evaluate the potential role of ras genes in the development of bladder cancer, this study analyzed the frequency of both amplification and mutation of c-Ha-ras-1 and c-Ki-ras-2, in 37 tumours, and the loss of c-Ha-ras-1 locus heterozygosity in 90 bladder tumours.

MATERIALS AND METHODS

PATIENTS AND TISSUES

The tumour tissues used in this study were obtained from the Urological Department of the Medical School Hospital (Besançon, France). C-Ha-ras-1 and c-Ki-ras-2 amplification and mutation were studied in 37 human transitional cell bladder cancers. C-Ha-ras–1 allelic loss was analyzed in 90 bladder cancers obtained from 73 patients: 57 patients with one tumour resection, 15 with one recidive and one with two recidives. Stage classification of the tumours studied was established according to the TNM (UICC 1978). The reference DNA was the WBC DNA obtained for each patient. The tumour tissues were frozen in liquid nitrogen immediately after surgical removal and stored in liquid nitrogen with WBC samples until they were processed.

HIGH-MOLECULAR-WEIGHT DNA PREPARATION

Tumour tissues were pulverized in liquid nitrogen. Tumour and WBC DNA extraction was carried out using Dykes (1988) modified method. In the purification step, Triton X-100 was substituted for SDS (sodium dodecyl sulfate), as Triton X-100 interferes with the binding of the nucleic acid on the chromatography resin (Qiagen, Coger, Paris, France). High-molecular-weight DNA was quantified by spectrophotometry at 260 nm. DNA purity was controlled by spectrophotometry at 280 nm to check the absence of protein contamination, and DNA quality was controlled by agarose gel electrophoresis followed by ethidium bromide visualization.

AMPLIFICATION ANALYSIS

For each sample, three DNA blots (10 μg) were performed. DNA was denatured in 0.5 M NaOH, 1.5 M NaCl at room temperature for 10 min and neutralized with 1 M Tris-base, 1.5 M NaCl pH 7.5. After blotting, nylon filters (Bioprobe System, Montreuil sous Bois, France) were baked for 2 h at 80°C in vacuo. Prehybridization and hybridization with the ^{32}P-labelled probes (10^4 cpm/cm) were performed as described by Reed (1986). Two DNA probes were used: c-Ha-ras-1, a 6.6 kb BamHI fragment of pUCEJ 6.6 (ATCC # 41028); c-Ki-ras-2, a 1.1-kb PstI/BamHI fragment of pSW11.1 (ATCC # 41027). The probes were radiolabelled by the Nick Translation procedure (specific activity: 3–5 × 10^7 cpm.μg^{-1}, Nick-translation kit, Boehringer Mannheim, Meylan, France).

MUTATION ANALYSIS

DNA amplification by polymerase chain reaction (PCR) followed by hybridization with mutation-specific synthetic oligonucleotide probes was used to detect and characterize mutational activations of the c-Ha-ras-1 and c-Ki-ras-2 genes in codons 12 and 61. Genomic DNA (1 μg) was submitted to 25 cycles of PCR amplification as described by Saiki et al (1985) and Verlaan de Vries et al (1986). To assess the amplification quality, an aliquot of the final reaction mixture (1/20) was submitted to an electrophoresis through a 12% native polyacrylamide gel (5 h, 5V/cm).

Aliquots of amplified DNA (1/10 of the final reaction mixture) were denatured and blotted to a nylon filter. Filters were prehybridized and hybridized in a mixture containing 3 M tetramethyl ammonium chloride as described by Verlaan de Vries et al (1986) and Farr et al (1988). Oligonucleotide probes (New England Nuclear Research Product) were ^{32}P-labelled by 3′-end-Tailing System (Bethesda Research Laboratory) and used at a 2×10^4 cpm/cm^2 concentration for hybridization (specific activity: 10^6 cpm.ng^{-1}).

C-HA-RAS-1 POLYMORPHISM ANALYSIS

DNA (10 µg) was restricted with BamHI (Boehringer Mannheim), electrophoresed through a 0.8% agarose gel for 17 h at 40 V, and blotted onto Hybond N^+ membranes (Amersham, Les Ulis, France) according to the method of Vacugene system (Pharmacia LKB, Saint Quentin en Yvelines, France). The membranes were prehybridized and hybridized according to the manufacturer's protocol. The DNA probe origin and radiolabelling are described above in the 'amplification analysis' section. The ^{32}P-labelled DNA probe was used at 0.25 ng/cm^2 of membrane for hybridization.

DENSITOMETRIC ANALYSIS

The filters were autoradiographed using X-OMAT film (Kodak) or Hyperfilm (Amersham) exposed with intensifying screen at −70°C. For amplification analysis, hybridization signals were quantified using a laser densitometer Ultroscan XL (Pharmacia LKB).

RESULTS

AMPLIFICATION AND MUTATION ANALYSIS

The degree of amplification was evaluated by the ratio (R) of the mean intensity (n = 3) of the hybridization signal for the tumour DNA to the mean intensity (n = 3) of the control WBC DNA. Out of the 37 tumours, no c-Ki-ras-2 amplification was detected and two tumours (5%) demonstrated c-Ha-ras-1 amplification ranging from 2.0 to 4.0 as shown in Figure 12.1. One c-Ha-ras-1-amplified tumour was a superficial tumour (pTa) with a low histological grade and a low mitotic index; the other amplified tumour was an invasive tumour (pT2) with a high histological grade.

C-Ha-ras-1 and c-Ki-ras-2 mutations were not detected in either codon 12 or codon 61 (Fig. 12.2).

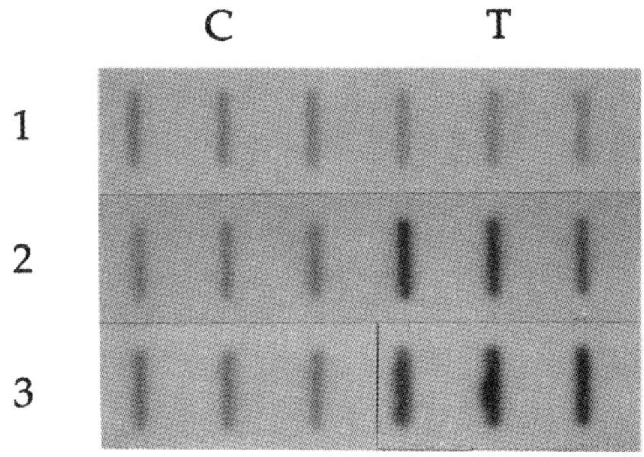

Fig. 12.1 Representative slot hybridization of c-Ha-ras-1 probe to control WBC (C) or tumour (T) DNA in human bladder cancer. Case 1: an unamplified tumour. Cases 2 and 3: two tumours with c-Ha-ras-1 amplification; the amplification levels are respectively ×3 and ×4

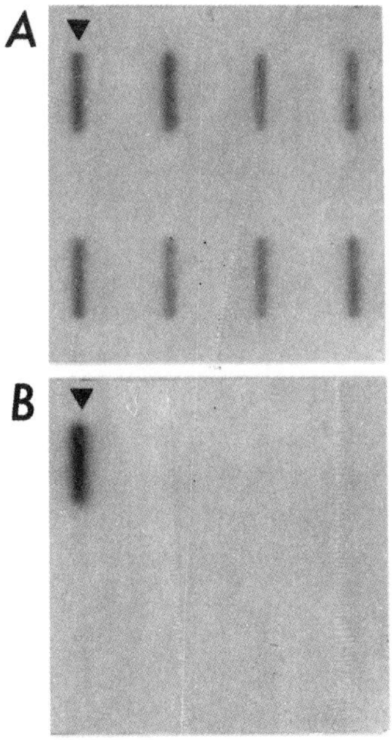

Fig. 12.2 Determination of point mutations in codon 12 of the c-Ha-ras-1 gene. Seven amplified DNA fragments have been blotted onto different filters. **A** Hybridization with the oligonucleotide probe wild type (codon 12: GGC encoding gly). **B** Hybridization with a mutation specific probe (codon 12: GTC encoding val). The sign (▼) identifies amplified DNA of T24 oncogene, positive control for gly→val mutation.

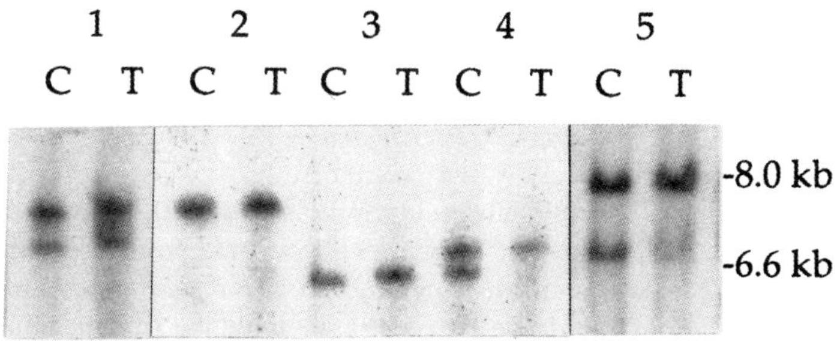

Fig. 12.3 Representative Southern hybridization of c-Ha-ras-1 probe to control WBC (C) or tumour (T) DNA in human bladder cancers. The size of BamHI restriction fragments are given in kilobase pairs (kb). Case 1: a heterozygous state in control and tumour tissue. Cases 2 and 3: a homozygous state. Case 4: a total loss of one allelic c-HA-ras-1 locus in the tumour tissue. Case 5: a partial loss of c-Ha-ras-1 locus in the tumour tissue.

C-HA-RAS-1 POLYMORPHISM

C-Ha-ras-1 polymorphism was obtained by hybridization of BamHI restricted WBC DNAs with 6.6-kb c-Ha-ras-1 fragment (Fig. 12.3). We found that 53% of these controls were heterozygous, i.e., two bands detected within the 6.6–8.0 kb range. The heterozygous state of the patients, determined in the WBC DNA, was not correlated with the stage of the tumours (superficial or pTa versus invasive or PT1 to pT4) as shown in Table 12.1.

We detected the four most frequent alleles, referred to as 'common' following the criteria of Krontiris et al (1985): a1 6.6 kb, a2 7.0 kb, a3 7.7 kb, a4 8.0 kb and the other BamHI digested fragments were considered as the rare alleles.

For the 39 heterozygous patients, the c-Ha-ras-1 polymorphism analysis was carried out in 50 tumour DNAs. A loss of one c-Has-ras-1 allele was observed in eight tumour DNAs (16%). This loss was partial in three tumours and total in five tumours. There was no c-Ha-ras-1 allelic loss in the other tumour DNAs.

Table 12.1 Relationship between tumour category (superficial or pTa versus invasive or pT1 to pT4) following the heterozygous or homozygous state determinated in the WBC DNA from the 73 patients (chi-2 test, $p > 0.05$).

Patient	Tumour category		
	Superficial	Invasive	NA*
Heterozygous	17	29	4
Homozygous	17	21	2

*NA = not applicable

DISCUSSION

Alterations by amplification or by point mutation of ras genes were seldom detected in human bladder cancers: only 5% of tumours exhibited c-Ha-ras-1 amplification without any association with a poor prognosis. These results agree with those reported by other authors: Hayashi et al (1983) reported c-Ha-ras-1 amplification in only one bladder carcinoma, and Fujita et al (1985) showed low frequency of ras gene mutations in urinary tract tumours. This was confirmed by most studies reviewed by Bos (1989). This author demonstrated, however, the high incidence of mutated ras genes in other tumour types, such as colonic, pancreatic, lung carcinoma and myeloid disorders. These reports and our results demonstrate that these alterations in ras genes are not the principal mechanism of activation in bladder cancers.

The VTR region length heterogenity was analyzed by Southern hybridization on genomic DNA digested with BamHI. This digestion provided different length fragments due to the repetitive unit of a 28-base-pair sequence. Our results on the c-Ha-ras–1 polymorphism revealed that 53% of cancer patients were heterozygous and that there was no significant correlation with a superficial or invasive stage of the tumours. A more detailed analysis of pathological stages is now in progress and it is thought that a correlation could exist between the heterozygous state and advanced tumour stage.

Overall, there was c-Has-ras-1 locus loss in 16% out of the 50 tumour DNAs from heterozygous patients. The loss of chromosome 11p heterozygosity in bladder tumours was observed in 39% of 23 tumours by Fearon et al (1985) and in 8% of 13 tumours by Pierotte et al (1989).

This study shows that c-Has-ras-1 RFLP is the most frequent ras gene alteration in bladder tumours. C-Ha-ras-1 RFLP suggests the potential involvement of loss of heterozygosity in human bladder cancers. A recessive gene, i.e., a tumour suppressor gene, could be located near the c-Ha-ras-1 locus.

To evaluate the deletion extent on chromosome 11p, the tumours with a loss of heterozygosity will be specifically analyzed. Other markers, on both sides of the c-Ha-ras-1 locus, will be studied.

REFERENCES

Bos J L 1989 *Ras* oncogenes in human cancer: a review. Cancer Res 49: 4682–4689
Capon D J, Chen E Y, Levinson A D et al 1983 Complete nucleotide sequences of the T24 human bladder carcinoma oncogene and its normal homologue. Nature 302: 33–37
Dykes D D 1988 The use of biotinylated DNA probe in parentage testing non isotopic labeling and non toxic extraction. Electrophoresis 9: 359–368
Farr C J, Saiki R K, Erlich H A et al 1988 Analysis of *ras* gene mutations in acute myeloid leukemia by polymerase chain reaction and oligonucleotide probes. Proc Nat Acad Sci USA 85: 1629–1633
Fearon E R, Feinberg A P, Hamilton S H et al 1985 Loss of genes on the short arm of chromosome 11 in bladder cancer. Nature 318: 377–380

Fujita J, Srivastava S K, Kraus M H, et al 1985 Frequency of molecular alterations affecting ras protooncogenes in human urinary tract tumors. Pro Nat Acad Sci USA 82: 3849-3853
Hayashi K, Kakizoe T, Sugimura T 1983 In vivo amplification and rearrangement of the c-Ha-ras–1 sequence in a human bladder carcinoma. Gann 74: 798–801
Krontiris T G, DiMartino N A, Colb et al 1985 Unique allelic restriction fragments of the human Ha-ras locus in leukocyte and tumour DNAs of cancer patients. Nature 313: 369–374
Nishimura S, Sekiya T 1987 Human cancer and cellular oncogenes. Biochem J 243: 313–327
Pierotti M A, Radice P, Lacerenza S 1989 Loss of 11p heterozygosity in human tumors of the urogenital tract. Cancer Cells 7: 279–282
Pulciani S, Santos E, Long L K et al 1985 Ras gene amplification and malignant transformation. Mol Cell Biol 5: 2836–2841
Reed K C 1986 Nucleic acid hybridizations with DNA bound to Zeta-probe membrane. Bio-Rad Bulletin 1234: 1–11
Saiki R K, Scharf S, Faloona F et al 1985 Enzymatic amplification of β globin genomic sequences and restriction site analysis for diagnosis of sickle cell anemia. Science 230: 1350–1354
UICC (Union Internationale Contre le Cancer) 1978 T.N.M. classification of malignant tumours, 3rd edn. International Union against Cancer, Geneva
Verlaan-De Vries M, Bogaard M E, Van Den Elst H et al 1986 A dot-blot screening procedure for mutated ras oncogenes using synthetic oligodeoxynucleotides. Gene 50: 313–32

13A. Amplification and expression of the c-erb B-2/neu and c-myc proto-oncogenes in bladder cancer and renal cell carcinoma

F. L. Gu J. C. Shen A. R. Zhou Z. L. Ge

INTRODUCTION

Abnormal activation of cellular proto-oncogenes has been proposed to play an important role in the initiation and development of human malignancies (Land et al 1983). Amplification and overexpression are important mechanisms of proto-oncogene activation (Schimke et al 1984). C-erb B-2 and c-myc are two members of the proto-oncogene family. The c-erb B-2-encoded p^{185} protein is related to, but distinct from, the epidermal growth factor receptor (EGFr) (Bargmann et al 1986). Amplification and overexpression of the human c-erb B–2 gene have been detected frequently in-human breast, ovarian and lung cancer (Zhou et al 1987, Slamon et al 1989, Schneider et al 1989). This may be a significant predictor of both overall survival and time to relapse in patients with breast cancer and ovarian cancer (Slamon et al 1987, Zhang et al 1989). Amplification and overexpression of proto-oncogene c-erb B-2 have been found in human bladder cancer (Haiyen et al 1990). Proto-oncogene c-myc was implicated in the control of cell growth and differentiation (Evan & Hancock 1985). The expression of the c-myc gene has been associated with a variety of human cancers (Salmon et al 1984). C-myc gene amplification occurred in only a small percentage of these tumours. Only a few studies have directly examined the expression of proto-oncogene c-myc in human renal cell carcinoma (Karthaus et al 1986). Bladder cancer and renal cell carcinoma are two of the most common human malignancies. We screened 20 bladder cancers, 22 renal cell carcinomas and human bladder cancer cell line BIU-87 (established in our institute) to detect c-erb B–2 gene, c-myc gene amplification and expression, and to research the relationship between amplification, expression and pathologic grade of tumour.

MATERIALS AND METHOD

Tissue samples.

Human bladder cancer and normal mucosa from 20 patients (cystectomy 8 cases, TUR-BT 12 cases), and human renal carcinoma and adjacent

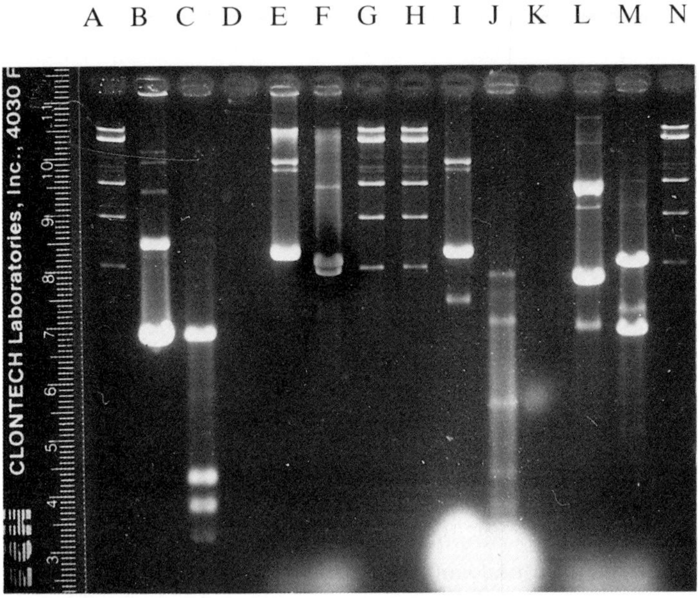

Fig. 13A.1 Electrophoresis of plasmid DNA. A,G,H and N mark DNA. B = pUC-β (4.6 kbp). C = pUC-β (4.6 kbp) EcoRI/BamHI 1.0 kbp. E = pSVerb B-2 (8.6 kbp). F = pSVerb B-2 (8.6 kbp) Hind III 4.6 kbp. I = PBR322myc (7.5 kbp). J = pBR322myc (7.5 kbp) EcoRI 1.0 kbp

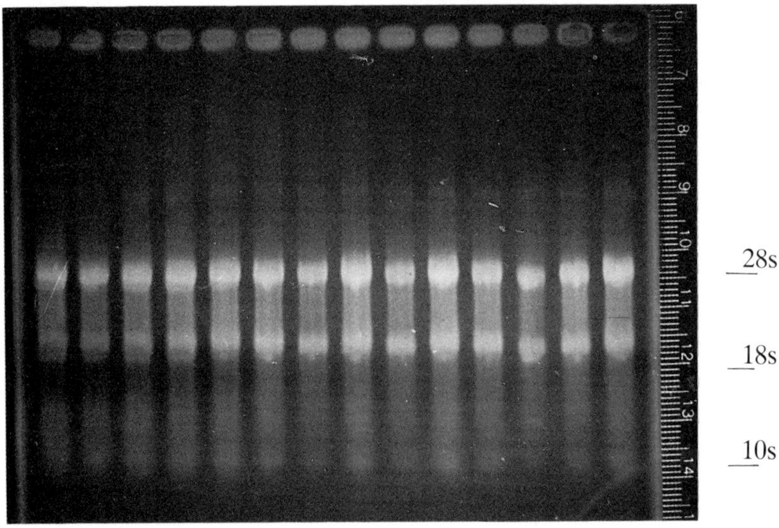

Fig. 13A.2 Electrophoresis of total RNA. Total RNAs were loaded on 1% agarose gel containing 2.2 formaldehyde.

normal tissue from 22 untreated patients (nephrectomy 22 cases) were used. Samples were obtained at the time of surgical resection at the Institute of Urology of Beijing Medical University and other hospitals in Beijing. The pathologic investigation was performed. All specimens were rapidly frozen in liquid nitrogen within 3 minutes and until the time of nucleic acid extraction.

BIU–87.

This human bladder cell line was established in our institute.

DNA probes.

We used pUC-t-β (4.6 kb), EcoRI/BamHI, and the β-globin gene (1.0 kb) as internal control. pSV erb B-2 (8.6 kb), HindIII and the erb B-2 gene probe 4.6 kb were kindly supplied by Dr T. Yamamoto, Tokyo University. pBR322 myc (7.5 kb) and EcoRI probe (1.0 kb) were obtained from the American Type Culture Collection. Plasmids were restricted with RE (Fig. 13A.1)

Isolation of DNA and Southern blot analysis.

Total DNA was extracted from tumour and normal tissue by the recommended method (Maniatis et al 1982). Ten μg of genomic DNA was digested with restriction endonuclease (EcoRI), electrophoresed on 0.8% agarose gels and transferred to nylon membrane. The nylon membrane was prehybridized and hybridized with nick-translated ^{32}P-labelled oncogene DNA probes (1–2 $\times$ 10^8 CPM μg^{-1}). The blots were washed for 20 min in 2 $\times$ SSC at room temperature and 60°C in 0.1 $\times$ SSC, 0.1% SDS with constant agitation, and exposed to Kodak film at -70°C for 1–3 days. The membranes were stripped off the c-erb B-2 signal and rehybridized with a human β-globin gene as internal control.

Isolation of RNA and Northern blot, slot blot analysis.

Total RNA was extracted by the guanidine isothiocyanate method (Cathala et al 1983). Electrophoresis was used to check the quality of total RNA (Fig. 13A.2). Poly (A^+) RNAs were selected from total RNAs by chromatography. mRNAs were denatured and electrophoresed on 1% agarose gels containing 2.2 M formaldehyde and transferred to a nitrocellulose (NC) filter. RNA samples were denatured and spotted on the NC filter. Filters were prehybridized and hybridized.

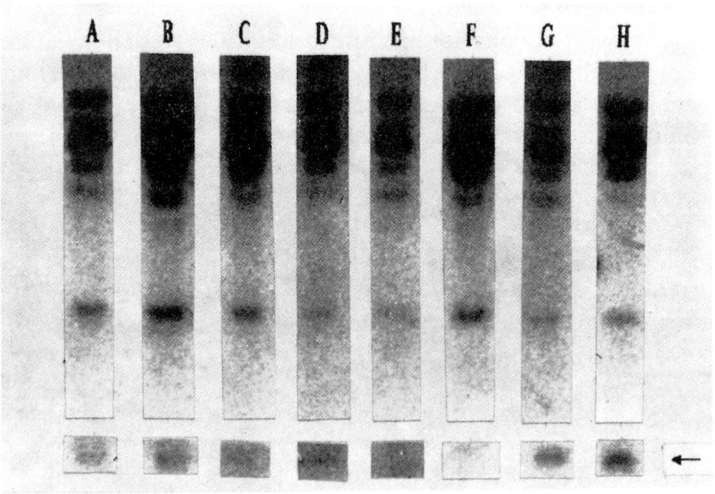

Fig. 13A.3 Analysis of the c-erb B-2 gene in human bladder cancer DNA. 10 µg of total DNA were prepared from normal bladder tissue (tracks A,C,E and G) and from tumour tissues (tracks B,D,F and H). DNA was digested to completion with EcoRI and run on an 0.8% agarose gel. The DNAs were transferred to nylon membrane and hybridized with c-erb B-2/ neu probe from pSVerb B-2 plasmid.

Table 13A.1 Association of c-erb B-2 gene amplification and nuclear grade of bladder cancer

Nuclear grade	Single copy	Amplified copies	$p(\chi^2$ test)
G_1	2	0	
G_2	10	0	< 0.05
G_3	4	4	

Table 13A.2 Association of c-erb B-2 gene overexpression and nuclear grade of bladder cancer.

Nuclear grade	No overexpression	Overexpression	$p(\chi^2)$
G_1	2	0	
G_2	4	6	0.05
G_3	2	6	

Table 13A.3 Association of c-myc gene overexpression and nuclear grade of renal cell carcinoma.

Nuclear grade	No overexpression	Overexpression	$p(\chi^2)$
G_1	2	0	
G_2	4	12	< 0.005
G_3	1	3	

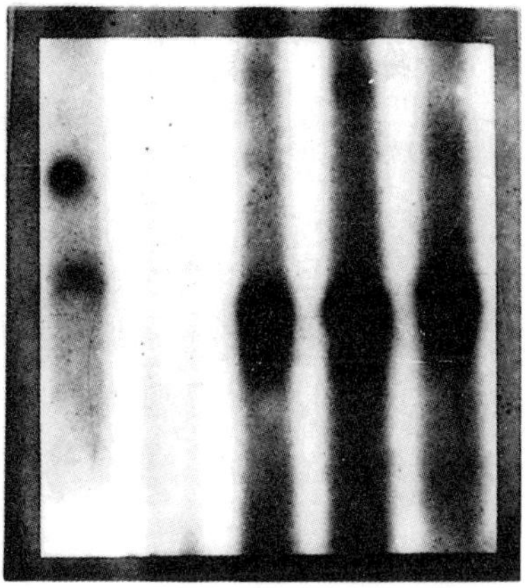

Fig. 13A.4 Northern blot: expression of the c-erb B-2 gene in human bladder cancer. Lane A: human bladder cancer cell line BIU-87. B: normal bladder tissue. C, D and E: bladder cancer tissue. Each lane contains 6 μg of poly(A)$^+$ RNA. Northern blot of bladder cancer shows an enhanced 4.8-kb c-erb B-2 band.

RESULTS

The amplification and expression of proto-oncogenes c-erb B-2 and c-myc were examined by Southern blot, Northern blot and slot blot in 20 bladder cancers, 22 renal cell carcinomas, and human bladder cancer cell line BIU-87.

HUMAN BLADDER CANCER

Southern blot analyses of DNAs from 20 bladder cancers showed 4 cases of c-erb B-2 gene amplification (2–6 fold) in carcinous tissue and none in normal tissue (Fig. 13A.3). Hybridization showed five bands for the c-erb B-2 gene (14.2, 8.0, 6.6, 4.8 and 1.8 kb) in human genomic DNA digested with EcoRI. Amplification of the c-erb B-2 gene was associated with poor nuclear grade of bladder cancer ($p < 0.05$) (Table 13A.1).

Northern blot and slot blot analyses demonstrated elevated levels of c-erb B-2 expression (2–10-fold) in 12 of 20 bladder cancers (Figs 13A.4 and 13A.5; Table 13A.2). Overexpression of c-erb B-2 was associated with poor nuclear grade of bladder cancer ($p < 0.05$). Amplification and overexpression of c-myc were not found in 20 bladder cancers.

RENAL CELL CARCINOMA

Twenty two renal cell carcinomas failed to amplify the c-erb B-2 and c-myc genes. Northern blot and slot blot analyses revealed that the levels of c-myc

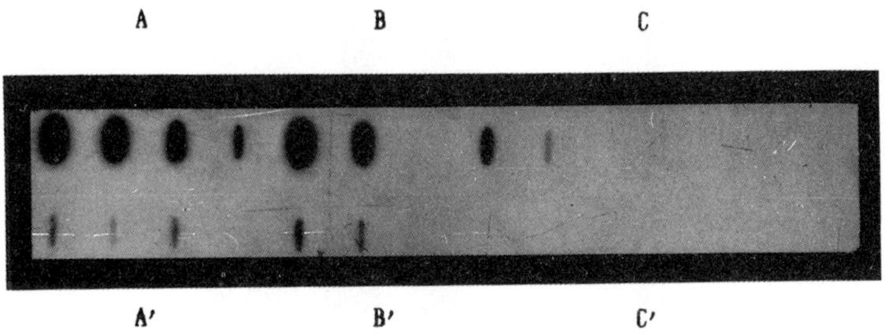

Fig. 13A.5 Slot blot hybridization of c-erb B-2 to RNA of human bladder cancer. A, B and C = bladder cancer. A′, B′ and C′ = normal bladder mucosa.

RNA increased (2–8-fold) in 15 of 22 renal cell carcinomas (Fig. 13A.6). Overexpression of the c-myc gene was associated with poor pathologic grade of renal cancer ($p < 0.005$; Table 13A.3).

BIU-87

Southern blot showed overexpression of the c-erb B-2 gene. Northern blot showed c-erb B-2 express a 4.8 kb mRNA band, and c-myc a 2.4 kb mRNA band.

DISCUSSION

Studies of the N-myc proto-oncogene were the first to show that there is a direct relationship between N-myc gene amplification and expression and

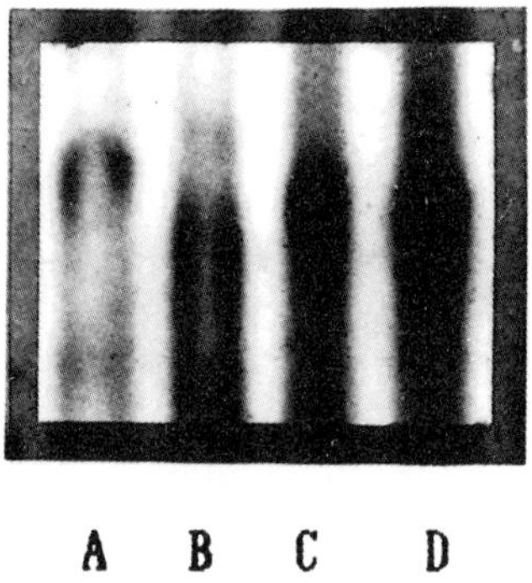

Fig. 13A.6 Northern blot: expression of the c-myc gene in human renal tissue. Lane A: normal renal tissue. B, C and D: renal cancer. Each lane contains 5 μ of poly(A)$^+$ RNA. mRNA of renal cell cancer shows an enhanced 2.4-kb c-myc band.

that these correlate with the stage of the disease and the survival of neuroblastoma patients (Brodeur et al 1934, Seeger et al 1985). Here, we investigated the possible involvement of the c-erb B-2 gene and c-myc gene in human bladder cancer and renal cell carcinoma development. We found that c-erb B-2 gene amplification occurred in 20% (4/20) of the bladder cancers. This value is more than those previously reported (Haiyen et al 1990). Sixty per cent (12/20) of the bladder cancers overexpressed the c-erb B2 gene. We think other mechanisms may also lead to an elevated level of expression. Amplification and overexpression of c-erb B-2 were associated with poor pathologic examination of human bladder cancer. We found that 68% (15/22) of the renal cell carcinomas overexpressed proto-oncogene c-myc. There is a relationship between c-myc gene overexpression and pathologic grade of renal cell carcinoma. We suggest that activation of c-erb B-2 may be involved in the development of human bladder cancer, and that c-myc is associated with renal cell carcinogenesis.

REFERENCES

Bargmann C I, Hung M C, Weinberg R A 1986 The neu oncogene encodes an epidermal growth factor receptor-related protein. Nature 319: 226–230

Brodeur G M, Seeger R C, Schwab M 1984 Amplification of N-myc in untreated human neuroblastomas correlates with advanced disease stage. Science (Washington DC) 224: 1121–1124

Cathala G, Savouret J F, Mendez 1983 A method for isolation of intact translationally active ribonucleic acid. DNA 2: 329–335

Evan G I, Hancock D C 1985 Studies on the interaction of the human c-myc protein with cell nuclei: $p^{62\text{-cmyc}}$ as a member of a discrete subset of nuclear protein. Cell 43: 253–261

Haiyen E Z, Xin Zhang, Andrew C et al 1990 Amplification and expression of the c-erb B-2/neu protooncogene in human bladder cancer. Mol Carcinog 3: 254–257

Karthaus H F M, Schalken J A, Feitz W F J et al 1986 Expression of the human fes cellular oncogene in renal cell tumor. Urol Res 14: 123–127

Land H, Parada L F, Weinberg R A et al 1983 Cellular oncogenes and multistep carcinogenesis. Science (Washington DC) 222: 771–778

Maniatis T, Fritsch E F, Sambrook J 1982 Molecular cloning. A laboratory manual. Cold Spring Harbor laboratory, New York

Salmon D J, dlkernion J B, Verma I M et al 1984 Expression of cellular oncogene in human malignancies. Science (Washington DC) 224: 256–262

Schimke R T 1984 Gene amplification, drug resistance and cancer. Cancer Res 44: 1735–1742

Schneider P M, Hung M C, Chiocca S M et al 1989 Differential expression of the c-erb B–2 gene in human small cell and non-small cell lung cancer. Cancer Res 49: 4968–4971

Seeger R C, Brodeur G M, Sath H 1985 Association with rapid progression of neuroblastomas. N Eng J Med 313: 1111–1116

Slamon D J, Clark G M, Wang S G et al 1987 Human breast cancer: correlation of relapse and survival with amplification of the HER–2/neu oncogene. Science 235: 177–182

Slamon D J, Godolphin W, Jones L A et al 1989 Studies of the HER–2/NEU protooncogene in human breast and ovarian cancer. Science 244: 707–712

Zhang X, Silva E, Gershehson D et al 1989 Amplification and rearrangement of c-erb B-2 protooncogenes in cancer of human female genital tract. Oncogene 4: 985–989

Zhou D, Battifora H, Yokota J et al 1987 Association of multiple copies of the c-erb B-2 oncogene with spread of breast cancer. Cancer Res 47: 6123–6125

13B. Induction of transforming growth factor alpha and oncogenes in bladder cancer

F. L. Gu   J. C. Shen   A. R. Zhou   Z. L. Ge

AIMS AND METHOD

Transforming growth factor α (TGFα) and oncogenes play important roles in abnormal growth of cancer. We investigated the expression and regulation of the TGFα gene, EGF/TGFα receptor and oncogenes in human bladder carcinoma tissues and bladder transitional cell carcinoma line BIU-87. TGFα mRNA and oncogene transcripts were detected with Northern and dot blotting. TGFα protein and receptor were detected by radioimmunoassay and radio-ligand binding assay, respectively.

RESULTS

In BIU-87 cells, TGFα mRNA was expressed and increased 3-fold at 4 hours, 2-fold at 8 hours after 12-0-teadecanoylphorbol-13-acetate (TPA) (100 ng/ml) treatment. TGFα (10 ng/ml, 8 hours) and EGF (10 ng/ml, 4 hours) increased TGFα mRNA by 1-3-fold.

TGFα protein in BIU-87 cells was detected after TPA(100 ng) treatment ($1.446 \pm 0.46\,ng/10^8$ cells, 4 hours; $0.726 \pm 0.19\,ng/10^8$ cells, 8 hours) but could not be detected in the untreated cells.

The amounts of BIU-87 cell-binding of ^{125}I-EGF were 28.8% and 27.7% of control at 4 hours and 8 hours after TPA (100 ng) treatment, respectively. The inhibition appears to involve decrease both in the numbers of EGFR and the affinity of EGFR for EGF.

c-myc, c-fos and v-erbB were expressed in BIU-87 cells. TPA increased the c-myc, c-fos and v-erbB mRNA.

We found the expression of TGFα gene, c-myc, c-fos and v-erbB in bladder cancer tissues. In contrast, no expression of these genes could be detected in normal bladder tissues.

CONCLUSION

The results suggest that TGFα and some oncogenes in bladder cancer may be regulated by some growth factors and tumour promoters. TGFα, c-myc, c-fos and v-erbB genes are responsible for the abnormal growth of bladder cancer.

REFERENCES

Carpenter G, Cohen S 1990 Epidermal growth factor receptor. J Bio Chem 265: 7709–7712

Ciardiello F, Kim N, Liscia D S et al 1989 mRNA expression of transforming growth factor in human breast carcinoma and its activity in effusions of breast cancer patients. J Natl Cancer Inst 81: 1165–1171

Derynck R 1988 Transforming growth factor $-\alpha$. Cell 54: 593–595

Derynck R, Goeddel D V, Ullrich A et al 1987 Synthesis of messenger RNAs for transforming growth factor α and β and the epidermal growth factor receptor by human tumors. Cancer Research 47: 707–712

Nowell P C 1986 Mechanisms of tumor progression. Cancer Research. 46: 3624–3628

Raymond W, Lee D C, Grisham J W et al 1989 Regulation of transforming growth factor $-\alpha$ mRNA expression in a chemically transformed rat hepatic epithelial cell line by phorbol ester and hormones. Cancer Research. 49: 3608–3612

Verma I M 1987 Regulation of c-*fos* oncogene expression. Cell 51: 513–517

14. Immunohistochemical expression of epidermal growth factor receptor and proto-oncogene erbB-2 in transitional cell carcinoma of the bladder

L. Nakopoulou A. Zervas V. Zolota D. Filaktopoulos C. Dimopoulos

INTRODUCTION

Transitional cell carcinoma (TCC) of the urinary bladder is the most common urinary tract tumour among men that leads to death (Morrison et al 1976). In the past 20 years, there has been no improvement in the management of TCC. At present, tumour grade and stage remain the best prognostic indices, but inter- and intra-observer inconsistency limit their clinical application (Ooms et al 1983, Abel et al 1988).

Recently, changes in expression of ABO system, growth factors and oncogenes, as well as the ploidy and aneuploidy of cancerous cells counted by flow cytometry (Emmott et al 1979, Fujita et al 1984, Neal et al 1985, de Vere White et al 1988) may represent useful markers in the prognosis of bladder cancer. More precisely, epidermal growth factor (EGF) is a low-molecular-weight polypeptide found in high concentration in human milk and urine (Oka & Orth 1983, Mattila et al 1986). The EGF receptor (EGFr) is a large molecule in the cell membrane. The EGF binding site faces the outside of the cell and the internal part of the receptor has protein kinase activity (Downward et al 1984). High levels of EGF expression have been identified in certain types of human malignant tumours (Cowley et al 1984, Gusterson et al 1985, Gullick et al 1986). Their presence in breast cancer is associated with a poor prognosis and has a negative relation with both oestrogen and progesterone receptors (Sainsbury et al 1985). Accordingly, there is accumulating evidence that overexpression of EGFr in bladder cancer correlates strongly with ominous prognostic factors (Berger et al 1987).

The c-erbB-2 gene – a recently identified proto-oncogene – encodes a

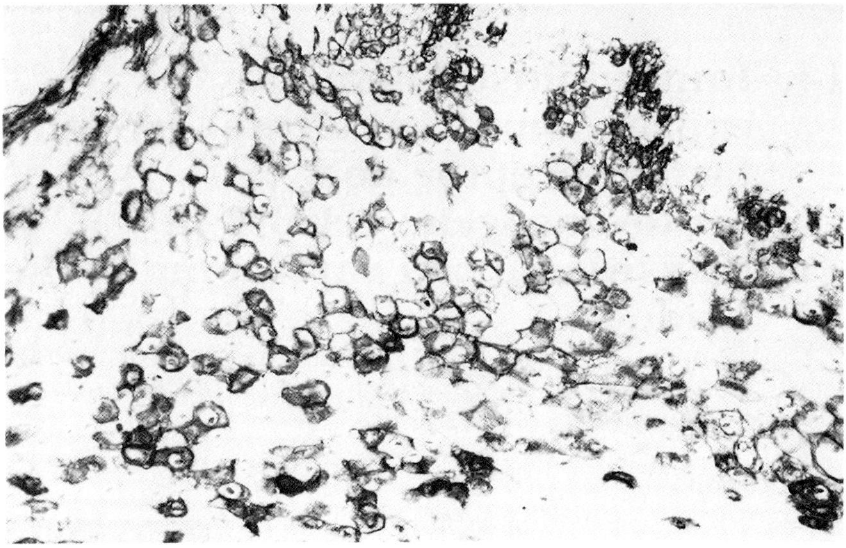

Fig. 14.1 Transitional cell carcinoma Grade III. Many cancerous cells stained positive with EGFr1 in the cytoplasm and (mainly) in the membrane (ABC × 300).

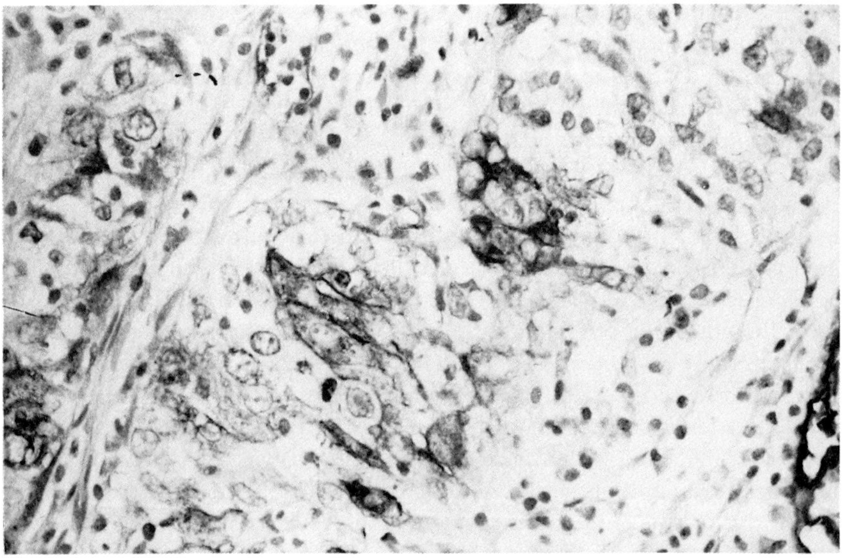

Fig. 14.2 Transitional cell carcinoma Grade III. Some tumour cells stained positive with EGFr1 in the cytoplasm and the membrane (ABC × 400).

185-kd transmembrane protein that has a homology to the EGFr, indicating that it too is a membrane receptor (Downward et al 1984). The amplification and/or overexpression of the c-erbB-2 oncogene has been shown to correlate with bad prognostic signs in women with breast cancer (Slamon et al 1987). However, the significance of overexpression of c-erbB-2 protein in bladder cancer is still controversial (Coombs et al 1991, Wright et al 1991).

In view of these findings, we have investigated the expression of both EGFr and c-erbB-2 gene in TCC specimens and correlated their expression with tumour grade and stage, and five-year survival.

MATERIAL AND METHODS

Our material consists of 24 urinary bladder cancerous tissues collected from patients operated on at Laikon General Hospital. Two of the tumours were classified as Grade I, 11 as Grade II, 10 as Grade III and two as Grade IV. Additionally, for of the tumours were stage T1, 12 stage T2, six stage T3, and four stage T4. The survival period ranged from one month to 64 months. Seven of the patients survived for more than five years. We performed the avidin-biotin immunohistochemical method (Hsu et al 1981) for both the EGFr and c-erbB-2 protein in 5 μm paraffin sections. The sections for the anti-EGFr monoclonal antibody were trypsinized (Trypsin Type II Sigma). Immunostaining for EGFr was carried out using a 1:80 dilution of the monoclonal antibody EGFr1 (66080-1 Biomakor), which recognizes the extracellular domain of the EGF receptor. C-erbB-2 protein was detected using the antibody 3B5 (Oncogene Sciences) raised against a synthetic peptide at the C-terminal (intramembranous) end of the c-erbB-2 gene product, at a dilution 1:20. Negative controls included omission of the primary antibody. As positive controls we used a breast carcinoma previously tested positive with both EGFr1 and anti-c-erbB-2 antibody.

RESULTS

Twelve of 24 bladder cancers were found to be positive with the monoclonal EGFr1 antibody. EGFr1 produced a combination of both cytoplasmic and membrane staining (Figs 14.1 and 14.2). The staining of tumour cells was highly heterogeneous in all the positive cases (Fig. 14.3). This heterogeneity took the form of negative staining of tumour masses that expressed 30–50% of the cells. Normal bladder urothelium was positive in five cases. In one case the staining was confined to the basal layer but in the rest of the cases it was distributed diffusely in the whole width of the urothelium. When the immunostaining was correlated with the histological grading, 2/2 Grade I tumours, 3/11 Grade II tumours, 6/10 Grade III and 1/1 Grade IV tumours were found to be positive (Table 14.1). With regard to the tumour stage, 1/4 T1 tumours, 4/12 T2, 5/6 T3 and 2/2 T4 tumours were also

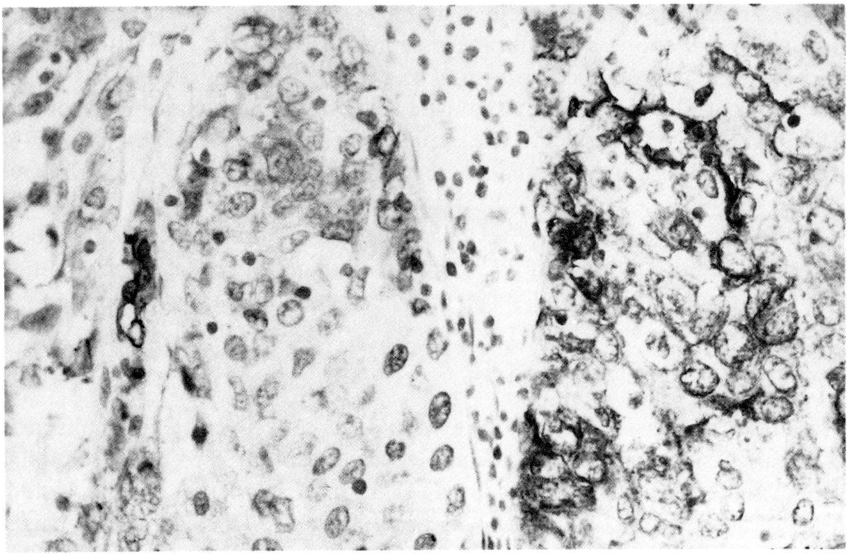

Fig. 14.3 Bladder cancer Grade III with focal expression of EGFr1 in many neoplastic cells (ABC × 400).

Table 14.1 Correlation of the expression of EGFr and c-erbB-2 protein with grade

Grade	No. of cases	EGFr	c-erbB-2
I	2	2	2
II	11	3	7
III	10	6	6
IV	1	1	1
Total	24	12(50%)	16(66%)

found to be positive (Table 14.2). Regarding the five-year survival, only one of the seven patients who survived more than five years, was strongly positive with EGFr1.

Most of our cases (16 of the 24 tumours) were positive for staining with 3B5, the anti-c-erbB-2 antibody. The staining was granular cytoplasmic and

Table 14.2 Correlation of the expression of EGFr and c-erbB-2 with stage

Stage	No. of cases	EGFr	c-erbB-2
T1	4	1	3
T2	12	4	7
T3	6	5	4
T4	2	2	2
Total	24	12(50%)	16(66%)

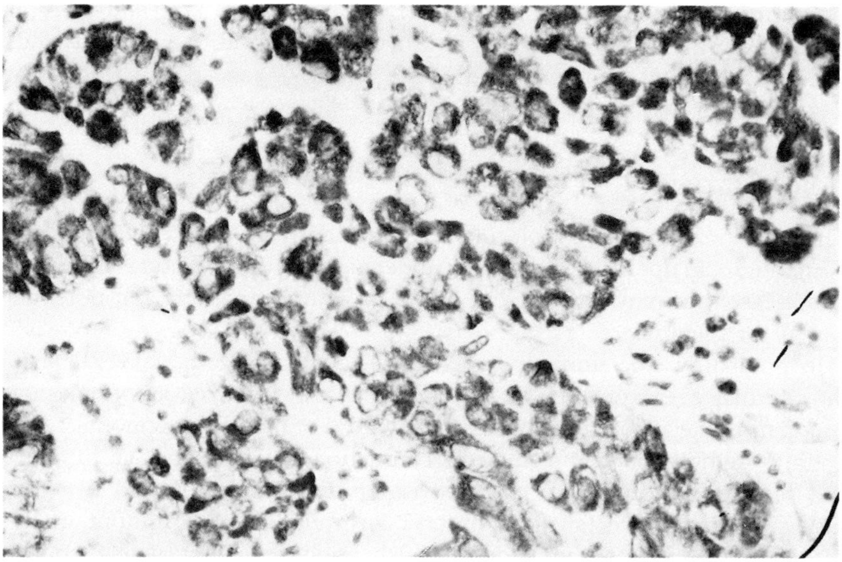

Fig. 14.4 Transitional cell carcinoma stained strongly positive with 3B5 antibody in many tumour cells in the cytoplasm and the membrane (ABC × 300).

membranous (Figs 14.4 and 14.5). In all of the positive cases the cancerous cells were almost homogeneously positive; very little heterogeneity was observed. We did not detect any significant association between c-erbB-2

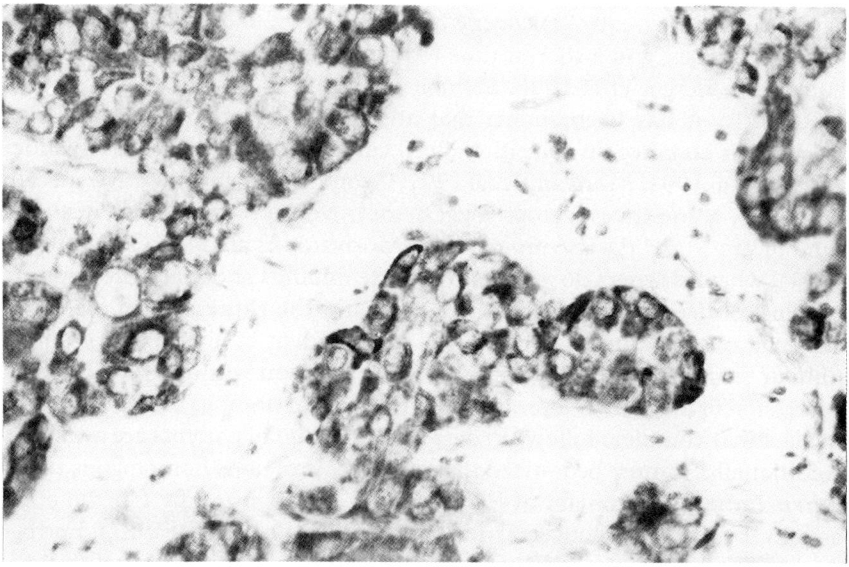

Fig. 14.5 The case shown in Figure 14.4, in higher power field (ABC × 400).

overexpression and grade or stage of the disease (Tables 14.1 and 14.2) or between c-erbB-2 overexpression and five-year survival. Additionally, our findings show that the expression of the c-erbB-2 gene product does not correlate with that of the EGFr.

DISCUSSION

The identification of the molecular events underlying urothelial cell transformation may not only expand our understanding of the natural history of the disease, but may also present useful prognostic markers and potential targets for therapy.

In our study, the immunocytochemical data, using the EGFr1 Mab, showed that overexpression of the EGFr can be visualized as cytoplasmic and membrane staining in approximately 50% of bladder carcinomas. Our findings demonstrated a significant correlation between positive tumours and bladder cancer stage, and between positive tumours and five-year survival, whereas we failed to observe any relation with tumour grade. These results are consistent with previously published papers which report a statistically significant correlation between positive tumours and invasion (Berger et al 1987, Wright et al 1991) but conflict with other recent data showing no relation with grade and stage (Moriyama et al 1911). However, the association of EGFr overexpression with five-year survival, observed in our work, supports the findings of Moriyama et al (1991).

The c-erb-2 is consistently amplified and/or overexpressed in a significant proportion of infiltrating breast carcinomas in a number of series (Slamon et al 1987, Berger et al 1988). In those patients, amplification and/or overexpression of the c-erb-2 oncogene has been shown to correlate with lymph node metastasis, and a shorter time to relapse and overall survival (Slamon et al 1987, Berger et al 1988, Slamon et al 1989).

Recently, it has been shown that amplification and overexpression of c-erbB-2 is common in transitional cell carcinomas of the urinary bladder (Wright et al 1991, Moriyama et al 1991, Coombs et al 1991). With respect to prognosis, some investigators suggest that overexpression correlates with tumour grade and disease progression (Moriyama et al 1991, Coombs et al 1991), whereas others do not confirm these findings and reach the opposite conclusion (Wright et al 1991). In our work, the expression of c-erbB-2, although observed in many cases, was independent of histological grading, tumour stage and five-year survival. No correlation was observed between expression of the c-erbB-2 product and EGFr. Our findings are reinforced by the fact that complete follow-up data for our group of patients are available. Additionally, it must be noticed that c-erbB-2 protein is homologous to the intramembranous domain of EGFr, which is recognized by F4, the other anti-EGFr antibody, not yet related to prognosis (Berger et al 1987). Further work based on larger number of cases is needed to determine the usefulness of c-erbB-2 and EGFr expression as prognostic markers in bladder cancer.

REFERENCES

Abel P O, Henderson D, Bennet M K et al 1988 Differing interpretations by pathologists of the pI category and grade of transitional cell cancer of the bladder. Br J Urol 62: 339–344

Berger M S, Greenfield C, Gullick W S et al 1987 Evaluation of epidermal growth factor receptors in bladder tumors. Br J Cancer 56: 533–537

Berger M S, Locher G W, Saurer et al 1988 Correlation of c-erbB-2 amplification and protein expression in human breast carcinoma with modal status and nuclear grading. Cancer Res. 48: 1238–1243

Coombs L M, Pigott D A, Sweeney E et al 1991 Amplification and over-expression of c-erbB-2 in transitional cell carcinoma of the urinary bladder. Br J Cancer 63: 601–608

Cowley G, Smith J A, Gusterson B et al 1984 The amount of EGF receptor is elevated in squamous cell carcinomas. In: Cancer cells. Vol. 1. The transformed phenotype, Cold Spring Harbor Laboratory, New York p5

de Vere White R N, Deitch A P, West B et al 1988 The predictive value of flow cytometric information in the clinical management of stage O (Ta) bladder cancer. J Urol 139: 279–282

Downward J, Yarden Y, Mayes E 1984 Close similarity of epidermal growth factor receptor and v-erb-B oncogene protein sequences. Nature 307: 521–527

Emmott R C, Javadpour N, Bergman S M et al 1979 Correlation of the cell surface antigens with stage and grade in cancer of the bladder. J Urol 121: 37–38

Fujita J, Yoshida O, Yuasa V 1984 Ha-ras oncogenes are activated by somatic alterations in human urinary tract tumors. Nature 309: 464–473

Gullick W J, Marsden J J, Whittle N et al 1986 Expression of epidermal growth factor receptors on human cervical, ovarian and vulval carcinomas. Cancer Res 46: 285–291

Gusterson B, Cowley G, McIlhinney J 1985 Evidence for increased epidermal growth factor receptors in human sarcomas. Int J Cancer 36: 689–695

Hsu S M, Rayne L, Fauger H 1981 Use of avidin-biotin-peroxidase complex (ABC) in immunoperoxidase techniques. J Histochem Cytochem 29: 577

Mattila A, Pasternack A, Vinikka L et al 1986 Subnormal concentrations of urinary epidermal growth factor in patients with kidney disease: J Clin Endocrinol Metab 62: 1180–1186

Moriyama M, Akiyama T, Yamamoto T et al 1991 Expression of c-erbB-2 gene product in urinary bladder cancer. J Urol 145: 423–427

Morrison A S, Cole P 1976 Epidemiology of bladder cancer. Urol Clin North Am 3: 13–25

Neal D E, Marsh C, Bennett M K et al 1985 Epidermal growth factor receptors in human bladder cancer: comparison of invasive and superficial tumors. Lancet i: 366–368

Oka Y, Orth D N 1983 Human plasma epidermal growth factor/B-urogastrone is associated with blood platelets. J Clin Invest 72: 249–259

Ooms, E C M, Anderson W A D, Alons C L et al 1983 Analysis of the performance of pathologists in the grading of bladder tumors. Hum Pathol 14: 140–148

Sainsbury J R C, Farndon J R, Sherbert V G et al 1985 Epidermal growth-factor receptors and estrogen receptors in human breast cancer. Lancet i: 364–366

Slamon D J, Clark G M, Wong S G et al 1987 Human breast cancer: correlation of relapse and survival with amplification of the HER–2/neu oncogene. Science 235: 177–182

Slamon D J, Godolphin W, Jones L A et al 1989 Studies of the HER–2/neu proto-oncogene in human breast and ovarian cancer. Science 244: 707–712

Wright C, Mellon, K, Johnston et al 1991 Expression of mutant p53, c-erbB-2 and the epidermal growth factor receptor in transitional cell carcinoma of the human urinary bladder. Br J Cancer 63: 967–970

15. Expression of multi-drug resistance gene product (P-glycoprotein) in normal urothelium and urothelial tumours

N. Shinohara M. Togashi I. Takeuchi T. Mori
M. Hamada Y. Asano B. Saitoh S. Nakanishi
T. Takamatsu A. Maru T. Koyanagi

ABSTRACT

Using the rabbit anti-human mdr polyclonal antibody (Ab-1; Oncogene Science), which was raised against the peptide in P-glycoprotein (P-GP)'s C-terminal cytoplasmic domain, we established the technique of P-GP staining in formalin-fixed, paraffin-embedded tissue sections, employing an avidine-biotin peroxidase method.

P-GP was detected in all of 14 cases with normal urothelium, suggesting that normal urothelium might possess multi-drug resistance with P-GP in order to protect itself from many exogenous chemical materials. We also investigated the expression of P-GP in 106 urothelial tumours (87 of bladder tumours, 10 of ureter tumours, and 9 of renal pelvic tumours). P-GP was expressed in 28 of 76 primary tumours and in 20 of 30 recurrent tumours. The expression of P-GP in recurrent tumours treated with adriamycin and its derivatives (15/18) is more frequent than that treated with others (5/12) ($p < 0.05$).

These data demonstrate that (1) urothelial tumours may arise from tissues normally expressing P-GP; (2) some of these tumours may possess intrinsic multi-drug resistance; and (3) pretreatment with adriamycin and its derivatives may induce P-GP in its negative urothelial tumours.

INTRODUCTION

Chemotherapeutic drug resistance by neoplastic cells appears to be a major clinical problem in the treatment of patients with a variety of tumours. The phenomenon of multi-drug resistance mdr further complicates the effective application of chemotherapeutic drugs in man. P-glycoprotein (P-GP), the product of the human mdr genes, is a transmembrane protein which acts by expelling several chemically unrelated chemotherapeutic agents from cyto-

Table 15.1 Characteristics of all specimens tested in this study

Normal urothelium (14)	Bladder (11)
	Ureter (2)
	Renal pelvis (1)
Urothelial tumours (106)	Bladder tumours (87):
	primary (58)
	recurrent (29)
	Ureter tumours (10):
	primary (9)
	recurrent (1)
	Renal pelvic tumours (9):
	primary (9)
	recurrent (0)

plasm, causing drug resistance (Kartner et al 1983, Moscow & Cowan 1988). Some of these agents, such as adriamycin and its derivatives, are frequently used for both intravesical and systemic chemotherapy of urothelial tumours. It is therefore of importance for clinical practice to elucidate whether P-GP actually is expressed by urothelial tumours without any prior exposure to adriamycin and its derivatives, and whether pretreatment with these agents induces P-GP in urothelial tumours or not.

We established the technique of P-GP staining in formalin-fixed, paraffin-embedded tissue sections, employing an avidine-biotin peroxidase method. Using this technique, we evaluated the expression of P-GP in both normal urothelium and urothelial tumours.

MATERIALS AND METHODS

Tissue specimens.

The specimens both of normal urothelium and of urothelial tumours were obtained from patients operated on at the University of Hokkaido Hospital and Jinyukai Urological Hospital. The specimens tested in this study are listed in Table 15.1

Antibodies.

For immunohistochemical study, we used the rabbit anti-human mdr polyclonal antibody (Ab-1; Oncogene Science). It was raised against the peptide (C,A,L,D,T,E,S,E,K,V,V,Q,E,A,L,D,K,A,R,E,G) in P-GP's C-terminal cytoplasmic domain. We used this polyclonal antibody at 2 μg/ml. As a negative control, an mdr antibody neutralized by preincubation with excess peptide immunogen mdr (Peptide–1, Oncogene Science) was used.

Immunohistochemical study.

Tissue specimens were fixed in 10% buffered formalin (pH 7.4) and embedded in paraffin. Serial sections were prepared from each specimen,

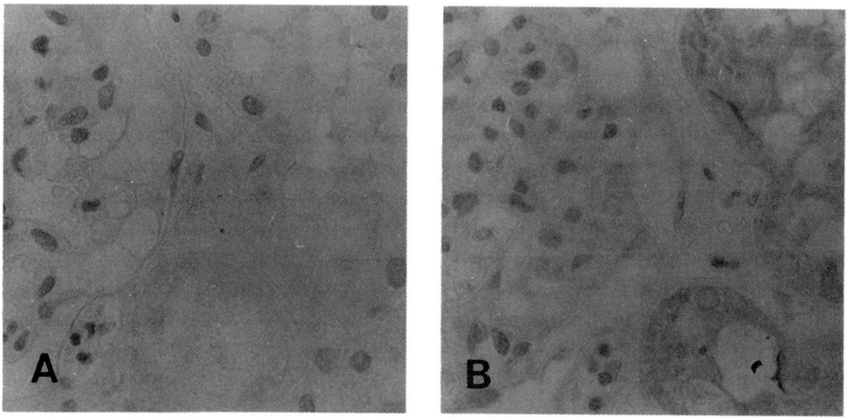

Fig. 15.1 Immunostaining of P-GP in normal kidney. **A** Negative control. **B** Positive reaction, predominant in the tubules of the kidney. ×400.

and then one from each was stained with haematoxylin and eosin for histopathologic diagnosis. The remaining sections were stained using a kit of the avidin-biotin-peroxidase complex (ABC) method (Vector) for immunohistochemical examination. These deparaffinized sections were treated with hydrogen peroxide to block endogenous peroxidase activity, incubated with 0.05% saponin solution, and then treated with normal goat serum to reduce nonspecific binding of the antibody. The sections were then incubated with anti-human mdr polyclonal antibody at 4°C overnight. Afterwards, the sections were treated first with biotinylated anti-rabbit serum, and second with horseradish peroxidase conjugated with avidin for 60 minutes at room temperature. Sections were then stained with diaminobenzidine followed by counter-staining with haematoxylin. A neutralized mdr antibody was used instead of a primary specific antibody for the negative control. Normal kidney and adrenal tissue, known to express a high level of P-GP, were used as a positive control (Sugawara et al 1988).

RESULTS

NORMAL TISSUES

Normal human kidney and urothelial tissues were tested for their reactivity with anti-human mdr polyclonal antibody. The tubules of the kidney, known to express a high level of P-GP, have a positive reaction (Fig. 15.1). Further, immunoreactivity to anti-mdr antibody was detected in all 14 samples of normal urothelium, including 11 samples of bladder mucosa, two samples of ureter mucosa (Fig. 15.2) and one sample of renal pelvis.

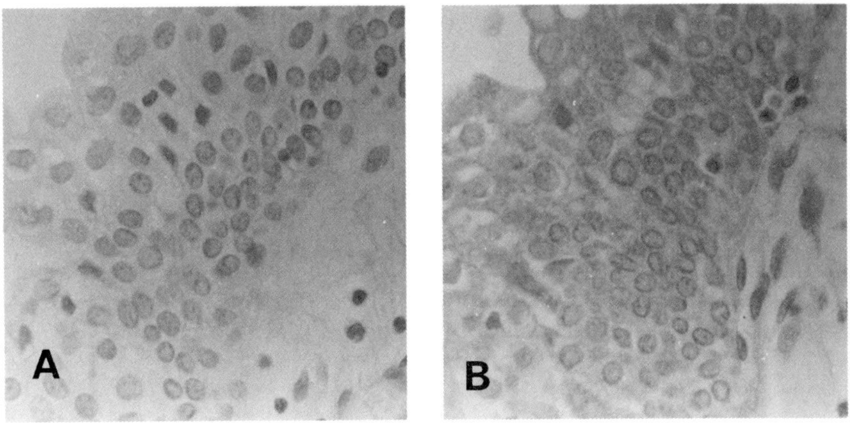

Fig. 15.2 Immunostaining of P-GP in normal ureter specimen. **A** Negative control. **B**. Positive reaction, predominant in the mucosa of ureter. ×400.

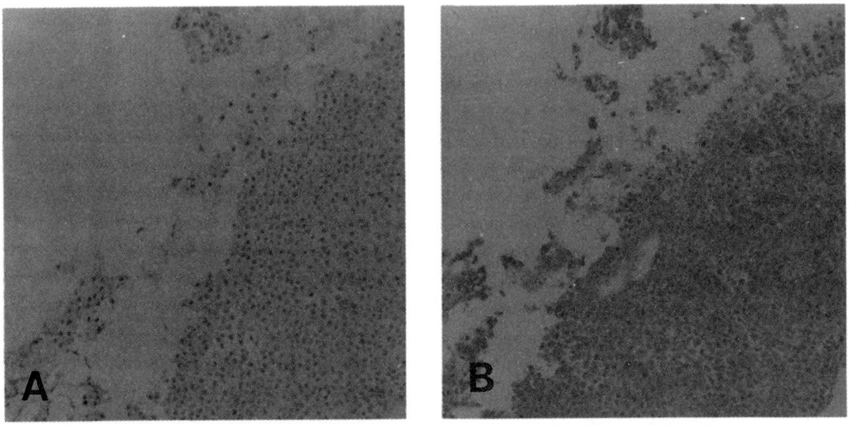

Fig. 15.3 Immunohistochemical detection of P-GP on untreated bladder cancer cells by anti-mdr polyclonal antibody. **A** Negative control. **B** Positive reaction. ×100.

Table 15.2 Immunohistochemical detection of P-GP expression in bladder, ureter, and renal pelvic tumours

	Reactivity of anti-mdr polyclonal antibody		
Tumour	+ve	−ve	Positive staining ratio
Bladder	42	45	48%
Ureter	3	7	30%
Renal pelvic	3	6	33%

Table 15.3 Expression of P-GP and the grade or urothelial tumour

Tumour grade	Reactivity of anti-mdr polyclonal antibody +ve	−ve	Positive staining ratio
G_0	2	3	40%
G_1	6	5	55%
G_2	25	29	46%
G_3	15	21	42%

TUMOUR SPECIMENS

The expression of P-GP in 106 urothelial tumours (87 of bladder tumours, 10 of ureter tumours, and 9 of renal pelvic tumours) was tested (Table 15.2 and Fig. 15.3). Positive immunostaining for P-GP was found in 42 of 87 bladder tumours (48%), 3 of 10 ureter tumours (30%), and 3 of 9 renal pelvic tumours (33%). The expression of P-GP was associated with histological grades of these tumours (Table 15.3). In terms of the expression of P-GP in primary and recurrent urothelial tumours, P-GP was found to be expressed in 28 of 76 primary tumours (37%) and in 20 of 30 recurrent tumours (67%). The expression of P-GP was more frequent in recurrent tumours than in primary tumours ($p < 0.01$; Table 15.4). The expression of P-GP was more frequent in recurrent tumours treated previously with adriamycin and its derivatives than in those without chemotherapy or with other treatments ($p < 0.05$; Table 15.5).

CONCLUSION

We reported the expression of P-GP in normal and malignant urothelial tissues, using a standard immunohistochemical technique.

Using anti-human mdr polyclonal antibody, we established the technique of P-GP staining in formalin-fixed, paraffin-embedded tissue sections, employing an avidin-biotin-peroxidase (ABC) method. As the paraffin sections are easy to use, a large number of clinical specimens can be effectively screened for the presence of the multidrug resistance and retrospective study is facilitated.

P-GP was detected in normal urothelium (bladder, ureter, and renal pelvis), suggesting that normal urothelium might possess multidrug resist-

Table 15.4 Immunohistochemical detection of P-GP expression in primary and recurrent urothelial tumours [$p < 0.01$ (chi-square test)]

Tumours	Reactivity of anti-mdr polyclonal antibody +ve	−ve	Positive staining ratio
Primary	28	48	37%
Recurrent	20	10	67%

Table 15.5 Comparison of P-GP expression with the effects of pretreatment in recurrent tumours*

Initial treatment	Reactivity of anti-mdr polyclonal antibody +ve	−ve	Positive staining ratio
Intravesical treatment with ADM and its derivatives	15	3	83%
No prior treatment or intravesical treatment with drugs other than ADM and its derivatives	5	7	42%

* $p < 0.05$ (chi-square test)

ance with P-GP in order to protect itself from many exogenous chemical materials including chemotherapeutic agents (adriamycin, vincristine, etc.).

P-GP was expressed by some of urothelial tumours (bladder, ureter, renal pelvis). These results indicate that urothelial tumours may arise from tissues normally expressing P-GP, and that some of these tumours may possess intrinsic multidrug resistance similar to that of colon and renal cell carcinoma.

The expression of P-GP was more frequent in recurrent tumours treated previously with adriamycin and its derivatives, than in those without chemotherapy or with other treatments. These results suggest that pretreatment with adriamycin and its derivatives induce P-GP in negative urothelial tumours or may select P-GP-positive urothelial tumours from primary tumours. Further study is necessary to clarify the situation.

REFERENCES

Kartner N, Riordan J R, Ling V 1983 Cell surface P-glycoprotein associated with multidrug resistance in mammalian cell lines. Science 221: 1285–1288

Moscow J A, Cowan K H 1988 Multidrug resistance. J Nat Cancer Inst 80: 14–20

Sugawara I, Kataoka I, Morishita Y et al 1988 Tissue distribution of P-glycoprotein encoded by a multidrug-resistant gene as revealed by a monoclonal antibody, MRK 16. Cancer Res 48: 1926–1929

16. Prostate cell proliferation and programmed death share an early molecular pathway regulated by androgens

R. Buttyan M. Schumer M. Colombel C. A. Olsson

INTRODUCTION

Differentiated prostatic epithelial cells are highly dependent on testosterone. Any manipulation that reduces the availability of this steroid will rapidly initiate an active death process in these cells, mechanistically referred to as *apoptosis* (Kerr & Searle 1973, Sanford et al 1984). As exemplified in the rat ventral prostate gland, one of the most suitable animal models for studying androgen-regulated apoptosis, this death process is extremely efficient, resulting in the elimination of up to 85% of the epithelial cells from the gland within the week after castration of a mature male rat (Bruchovsky et al 1975, English et al 1989). Since this is also the process by which androgen-deprivation therapy effects tumour regression in human prostate cancers, it is important that we fully understand the molecular basis for androgen action in cell death so that novel therapeutic approaches can be developed for this disease that is escalating in occurrence and increasing morbidity in the male population.

In contrast to *necrosis*, the more classically understood form of passive cell death, apoptosis is more similar to other genetically-driven cell processes such as proliferation and differentiation. Like apoptosis, each of these latter activities are initiated by changes in the cellular growth factor (or cytokine) environment, each requires energy expenditure by the cell, and each process is accompanied by definable morphologic changes in cell structure unrelated to simple degradation phenomenon. Because of these similarities, apoptosis is also referred to as a *programmed cell death*. Early experiments by Lee & Grayhack and their colleagues demonstrated that castration-induced prostate apoptosis can be suppressed by protein- and RNA-synthesis inhibitors (Stanisic et al 1978, Lee 1981). Therefore, again similar to other cell activities, androgen-regulated prostate cell apoptosis requires the ongoing synthesis of RNA and protein. Based on this observation, we can surmise that some protein(s) made by the prostate cell *after castration* is needed for the cell to die.

It has already been possible to identify a number of unique gene products synthesized by androgen-deprived prostate cells undergoing apoptosis. These products include sulphated glycoprotein-2 (Bandyk et al 1989), the Yb_1 subunit of glutathione S-transferase (Chang et al 1987) and cathepsin-D (Sensibar et al 1990). To date, none of these gene products has been proven lethal to the cell that synthesizes them. Rather, it has been hypothesized that they might play a role in protection of surrounding tissues from inflammatory response or in degradation of apoptotic remnants (Buttyan 1991). One unique observation, however, has been that prostate cells undergo a 'reactive cascade' of gene activity early after castration. This cascade consists of an early induction of mRNA encoded by the proto-oncogene c-fos gene, a later induction of c-myc mRNA and transcripts encoding heat-shock 70 K protein (Buttyan et al 1988). The reactive cascade has been extensively described in cultured cells stimulated to proliferate (Muller et al 1984), in regenerating organs such as the liver following partial hepatectomy (Thompson et al 1986) and, as we have shown earlier, also in prostatic epithelial cells stimulated to regrow by testosterone replenishment (Katz et al 1989).

This observation seems to be a paradox: why would cells undergoing two extremely different processes (apoptosis and proliferation) share the same early genetic response? It is also initially difficult to understand why two proto-oncogenes such as fos and myc, both of which are known to be strong promoters of cellular proliferation, might be induced during a process that leads only to cell death. Moreover, both apoptosis and proliferation share certain other physiological characteristics during their progression. Both our own laboratory and others have reported that prostate apoptosis can be suppressed by drugs that block membrane calcium channels (Connor et al 1988; Kyprianou et al 1988). These observations indicate that acute Ca^{2+} ion fluxes are important for this androgen-regulated apoptosis in the same manner that Ca^{2+} ion fluxes are required for cellular proliferation (Durham & Walton 1982). Coincidentally, it was recently demonstrated that these same calcium channel antagonists are potent suppressors of prostate cell proliferation (Batra et al 1991). Therefore, we believe that this series of observations implies that apoptosis and proliferation are related processes and strongly suggests the possibility that prostate apoptosis is initiated by the inappropriate entry of differentiated epithelial cells into the cell cycle. As a test of this hypothesis, we have begun to evaluate the activity of other proliferative markers, including tyrosine phosphorylation, ornithine decarboxylase expression and bromodeoxyuridine incorporation in prostate cells after castration. The results of our study, presented here, support our hypothesis, and provide new insights into the molecular mechanism of programmed death in the prostate, and in other organs.

TYROSINE PHOSPHORYLATION IN THE REGRESSING RAT VENTRAL PROSTATE GLAND

Phosphorylation of tyrosine residues on proteins is known to play a key role in mammalian cell growth regulation. This principle was first demonstrated in studies of the mechanism by which polypeptide growth factors initiate a proliferation response. Growth factors, such as epidermal growth factor (EGF), stimulate cell proliferation after binding to their specific receptor protein on the cell surface. In many cases, this binding promotes a conformational change in the receptor protein that results in the acquisition of tyrosine kinase activity by the cytoplasmic domain of the receptor (Di Fiore et al 1990). The activated growth factor receptor is then capable of phosphorylating tyrosine residues on adjacent membrane proteins, and on certain cytoplasmic proteins (Ellis et al 1990), and is also capable of autophosphorylating its own tyrosine residues (Naldini et al 1991) if in conformational proximity to the kinase domain. While the end point of tyrosine-phosphate mediated signal transduction is not yet clear, there is ample evidence, based on mutational analysis (Fantl et al 1989) and on the use of tyrosine-kinase inhibitors (Yoneda et al 1991) that this tyrosine kinase activity is necessary for cell cycle progression. It is also of note that several of the known oncogenes, exemplified by met (Naldini et al 1991) and kit (Rolink et al 1991), are modified growth factor receptors with constitutively active tyrosine kinase domains.

In an experiment designed to evaluate whether tyrosine kinase activity might increase during prostatic apoptosis, we utilized a Western-blot procedure to detect proteins with phosphorylated tyrosine residues (P-tyr proteins) in the normal and regressing rat ventral prostate gland. In an initial experiment, the ventral prostate gland was recovered from an adult male rat and from age-matched rats at progressive intervals after castration (6, 12, 18, 24, 36, 48, 60 and 72 h). These glands were homogenized in a protein-extraction buffer, then aliquots containing 100 μg of protein from each specimen were electrophoresed in adjacent lanes on SDS-polyacrylamide gels. The proteins in the gel were transferred to nitrocellulose with an electroelution device. This Western blot was probed with a rabbit polyclonal anti-tyrosine antibody (Upstate Biotechnology, Inc.) then stained with alkaline-phosphatase secondary antibodies and substrate to detect tyrosine-phosphorylated proteins. As shown in Figure 16.1, the control rat ventral prostate exhibited two prominent bands of reactivity with the antibody at approximately 40 kD, and several bands below this region. While these same bands were present in all extracts obtained from post-castrate prostate glands, there were at least two additional prominent bands of higher molecular weight (approximately 105 kD) in most of these later specimens. These high-molecular-weight bands appeared in a time-dependent fashion, being initially detectable at 6 hours after castration, very abundant at 24 hours after castration and subsequently declining in con-

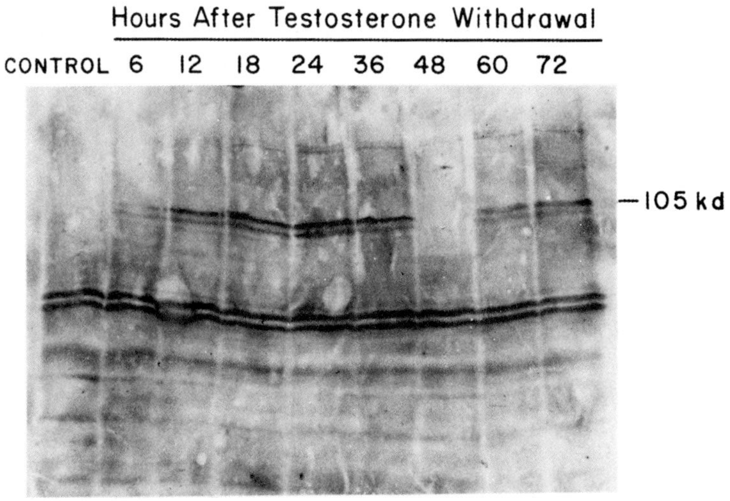

Fig. 16.1 Western blot detection of tyrosine-phosphorylated proteins in the regressing rat ventral prostate gland. Ventral prostate tissue from an adult rat (control) or from rats at sequential times after castration (Hours After Testosterone Withdrawal) were frozen, pulverized and extracted by homogenization in a buffer containing 50 mM Tris-HC1, pH 7.2, 1 mM EDTA, 0.5% Triton X–100 with 1 mM PMSF, 1 mM leupeptin and 1 mM aprotinin to inhibit endogenous proteases. Extracts were centrifuged at 12 000 × G for 15 min to pellet nuclear debris and the supernatants were removed and quantitated for protein concentration by the modified Bradford assay supplied by Sigma Chemical Co., St. Louis, MO, USA. Aliquots containing 100 µg protein were solubilized in sodium dodecyl sulphate-polyacrylamide gel (SDS-PAGE) buffer as proscribed by Laemmli (1970), then electrophoresed in consecutive lanes on a 12% SDS-acrylamide gel. Prestained molecular weight markers were co-electrophoresed in an adjacent lane. Proteins in the gel were transferred to nitrocellulose by electroelution at 150 mA overnight. The Western blot was blocked with a 10% solution of powdered milk in 50 mM Tris-HC1, pH 7.2, 0.15 M sodium chloride and 10 mM sodium borate (TBS). Following incubation with the primary polyclonal rabbit anti-tyrosine-phosphate antibody (Upstate Biochemical, Inc., Lake Placid, NY, USA), the blot was washed extensively then incubated with biotinylated secondary goat anti-rabbit IgG. Reactivity was visualized with the ABC-staining reagents in the Vectastain immunocytochemistry kit. Results shown above demonstrate the appearance of several high-molecular-weight bands reactive to the primary anti-tyrosine phosphate antibody only after castration.

centration. It was also notable that the 48-hour castrated specimen lacked the reactive bands above 44 kD.

In order to determine the reproducibility of this pattern and whether it was a function of the operational stress, we recovered individual ventral prostate glands from three rats that were castrated and had testosterone immediately replenished with a time-release subcutaneous implant (1 mg/day release, Innovative Research, Inc., Toledo, Ohio, USA) (Control Testosterone-Stimulated); from three rats at 24 hours after castration (Testosterone Withdrawn 24 hours); and from three rats at 48 hours castration (Testosterone Withdrawn 48 hours). Each specimen was processed individually for protein extraction, and aliquots containing 100 µg of protein were electrophoresed in adjacent lanes of an SDS-PAGE and blotted as

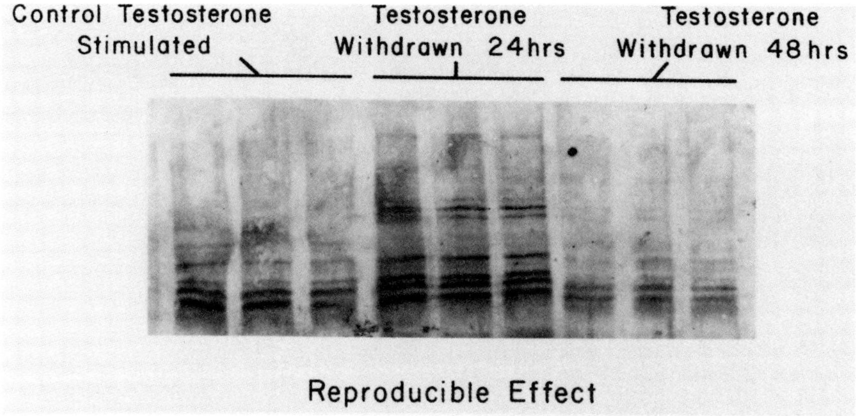

Fig. 16.2 Reproducible induction of novel tyrosine-phosphorylated proteins in the 24-hour castrated rat ventral prostate gland. Protein extracts were made from three individual ventral prostate glands from sham-castrated rats (Control Testosterone Stimulated); from three glands at 24 hours after castration, and from three glands at 48 hours after castration. Aliquots containing 100 μg of protein were electrophoresed in adjacent lanes of a 12% SDS-PAGE gel, then transferred to a nitrocellulose filter to produce a Western blot. The Western blot was probed for tyrosine-phosphorylated proteins using the procedure described in Figure 16.1. The results reproduce our original experiment and demonstrate the appearance of a series of tyrosine-phosphorylated protein bands in the high-molecular-weight region of all protein extracts from 24-hour castrated rat ventral prostate glands.

in the previous experiment. Immunodetection with the anti-tyrosine phosphate antibodies demonstrated results (Fig. 16.2) similar to the previous experiment; i.e. a series of high-molecular-weight bands present only in extracts made from 24-hour castrated prostates and not in the control (sham-castrated) extracts nor in the extracts from 48-hour castrates. These results reproduce our initial findings and show that novel tyrosine-phosphorylated proteins can be detected in prostate tissue during the early period following castration.

It is of interest to note that at least two of the bands identified by the monoclonal anti-phosphotyrosine antibody appear to be more specific for apoptosis than for proliferation. In Figure 16.3, we present results from an experiment designed to compare P-tyr protein patterns in highly proliferating, highly apoptotic, or homeostatic rat ventral prostate tissue. Rats were castrated and prostate regression was allowed to occur for 8 days. At this time, time-release testosterone pellets were implanted subcutaneously, thus stimulating ventral prostate regrowth. According to several studies on this system, proliferation of prostatic epithelial cells reaches a peak at 3 days following T-repletion. Tissue was recovered at this time (highly proliferative) and again at 8 days after repletion, by which time the prostate gland has recovered its normal size and is no longer growing (homeostatic tissue). At

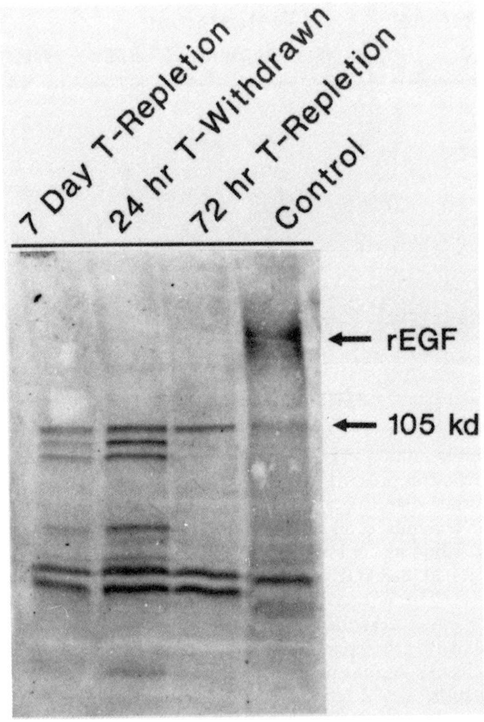

Fig. 16.3 Comparison of tyrosine-phosphorylated proteins in rat ventral prostate glands containing mainly proliferative or mainly apoptotic prostate cells. Eight-day castrated rats received subcutaneous implants of time-release testosterone pellets (25 mg released over 21 days; Innovative Research, Inc., Toledo, OH, U.S.A.) to stimulate regrowth of the ventral prostate gland. At three days, one group was sacrificed to obtain proliferative tissue (72-hour T-repletion) while others were harvested seven days after implantation to obtain homeostatic tissue (7-day T-repletion). At seven days after repletion, an additional group was harvested 24 hours after removal of the testosterone pellet (24-hour T-withdrawn) to provide highly apoptotic tissue. All tissues were extracted for protein and aliquots containing 100 μg were electrophoresed in adjacent lanes of a 12% SDS-PAGE in addition to an extract of EGF-stimulated WI38 cells (Upstate Biotechnology, Inc., Lake Placid, NY, USA) a source of tyrosine-phosphorylated EGF receptor (EGFr, 180 kD). The proteins in the gel were transferred to a nitrocellulose filter and the Western blot was probed for tyrosine-phosphorylated proteins. Results demonstrate two extra high-molecular-weight bands present in the highly apoptotic tissue extract compared to the highly proliferative tissue extract.

this time, the T-pellet implants were removed from remaining rats, and ventral prostate tissue was recovered from these T-depleted rats at 24 hours after removal (highly apoptotic). Protein extracts made from these tissues were analyzed for P-tyr patterns. As shown in Figure 16.3, highly proliferative prostate tissue had a band reactive to anti-P-tyr at 105 kD, while highly apoptotic tissue also demonstrates this band, in addition to two bands of lower molecular weight (approximately 100 and 95 kD) which appear with intensity. In contrast, the homeostatic tissue had light bands at all of these sites, potentially representing the homeostatic state of low levels of proliferation equalling low levels of apoptosis.

INDUCTION OF ORNITHINE DECARBOXYLASE mRNA DURING RAT VENTRAL PROSTATE REGRESSION

Another proliferative marker of the mammalian cell is the expression of the ornithine decarboxylase (ODC) gene. This gene encodes an enzyme that catalyzes the conversion of ornithine to putrescine, and is the first, and apparently rate-controlling, enzyme in polyamine biosynthesis (Williams-Ashman & Canellakis 1979). Perhaps because it is mainly required during DNA synthesis in S-phase, ODC expression is highly regulated during the cell cycle. Using a mouse ODC cDNA probe (Hickok et al 1986), provided by Dr. Olli Janne (Rockefeller University, New york, NY), we hybridized a Northern blot containing a series of mRNAs extracted from rat ventral prostate glands at sequential intervals after castration. The autoradiograph showing the results of this hybridization (Fig. 16.4) demonstrates that the 2.2-kb transcript homologous to our probe was undetectable in control rat ventral prostate mRNA and in sham-castrated rats at 3 days following the sham operation. ODC mRNA was present in ventral prostate mRNA at 12, 24 and 72 hours after castration, however. Densitometric quantitation of the autoradiograph allows us to estimate an 8-fold elevation in the expression of this mRNA within the first 24 hours after castration. Therefore, ODC expression, a distinct marker of proliferation, is also induced in the ventral prostate gland during the early period following castration. Since this is the time period when most of the prostate epithelial cells are entering apoptosis, we believe that early ODC induction is also a marker of this phenomenon.

BROMODEOXYURIDINE INCORPORATION IN THE VENTRAL PROSTATE GLAND AFTER CASTRATION

As we have discussed, apoptotic prostate demonstrates several characteristics that we once associated exclusively with cells undergoing proliferation. These characteristics include the induction of a proto-oncogene cascade, induction of ODC expression and the appearance of novel tyrosine-phosphorylated proteins. As a more functional test of the relationship between apoptosis and proliferation, we also studied whether apoptotic prostate epithelial cells incorporate bromodeoxyuridine (BrdU) into their DNA prior to their elimination from the gland. BrdU is a thymidine analogue that can be scavenged with the aid of cellular thymidine kinase and subsequently utilized for DNA synthesis in a replicating cell. This analogue can be detected with a simple immunocytochemical procedure and is being increasingly used to identify proliferative cells in both in vivo and in vitro

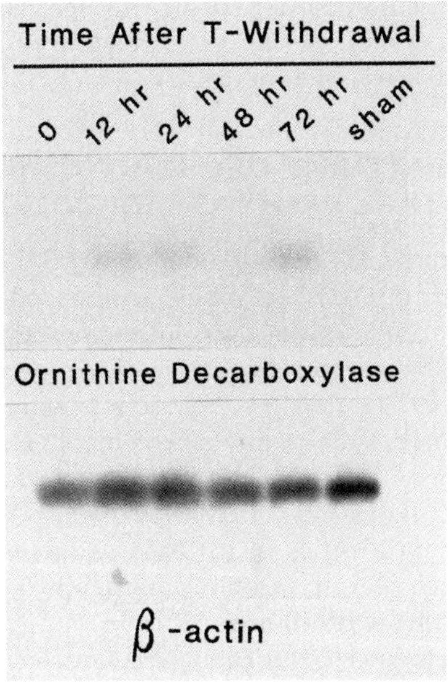

Fig. 16.4 Expression of mRNA encoding ornithine decarboxylase in the regressing rat ventral prostate gland. Poly $(A)^+$ mRNA was extracted from unoperated rat ventral prostate glands (0) or from ventral prostate glands obtained at sequential intervals after castration, as well as from 24-hour sham-castrated rats by the method described by Buttyan et al (1988). Aliquots containing 5μg of mRNA were electrophoresed on a 1.2% formaldehyde agarose gel as described. The RNA was blotted onto Nytran nylon filter paper (Schleicher and Schuell, Inc., Keene, NH, U.S.A.) to produce a Northern blot. The blot was hybridized to the cDNA probe for ODC (Hickok et al 1986) labelled with ^{32}P as described (Buttyan et al 1988). The hybridized blot was exposed to Kodak XAR–5 X-ray film to autoradiograph, and the Northern blot was then cleaned and rehybridized to a cDNA probe for β-actin. Densitometry of the autoradiographs on a Molecular Dynamics Scanning Densitometry provided an estimate of eight-fold induction in ODC expression by 24 hours after castration.

systems. To identify proliferating cells, BrdU is administered to the rat in an i.p. solution. Tissues can be harvested at times after this treatment, fixed and embedded, thin-sectioned then immunostained for BrdU incorporation into nuclear DNA. We found that there was very little BrdU incorporation in a normal adult rat ventral prostate gland following a 6-hour pulse of BrdU (less than one epithelial nucleus labelled per prostatic duct) and this is consistent with the low rate of proliferation previously assigned to this tissue. In startling contrast (Fig. 16.5), an equivalent pulse of BrdU given to a 60-hour castrate rat labels numerous epithelial cell nuclei within the gland. Since there is no mitosis detected in the post-castrate ventral prostate, we believe that BrdU incorporation is a prelude to apoptosis, that this incorporation is indicative of active DNA synthesis in the apoptotic cell and

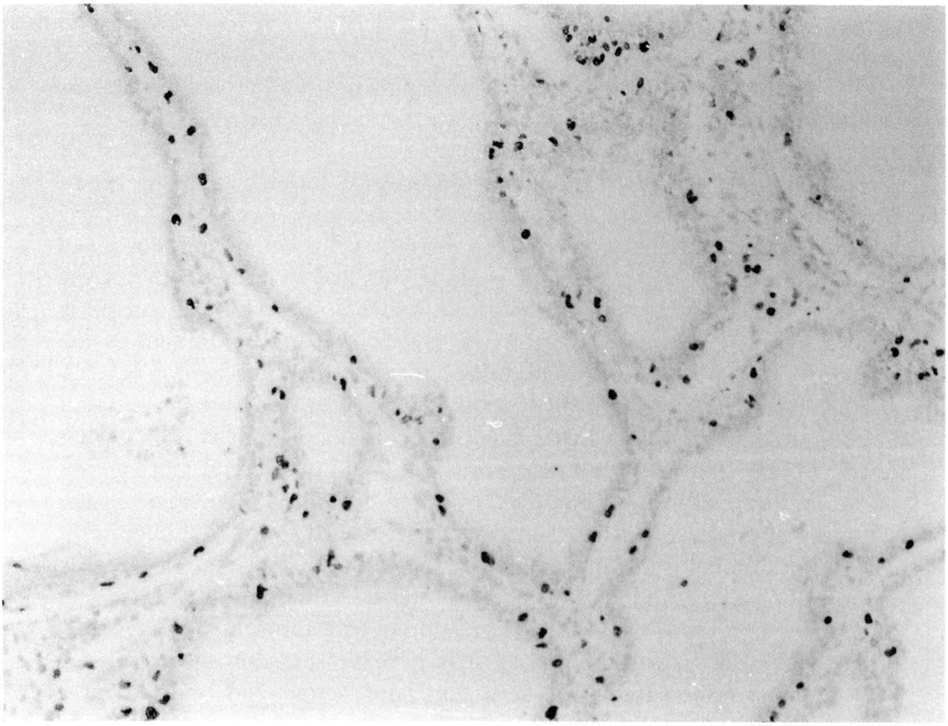

Fig. 16.5 Photomicrograph of BrdU-labelled epithelium nuclei in a regressing rat ventral prostate gland. At 60 hours after castration, a rat received an intraperitoneal solution of BrdU (50 mg/kg). Six hours later, the rat was sacrificed, the ventral prostate was recovered, fixed in neutral formalin, dehydrated and embedded in paraffin. A 3-μm section was immunostained for BrdU incorporation by the method of Schutte et al (1987). Magnification (200×) shows numerous immunoperoxidase-labelled nuclei demonstrating extensive DNA synthesis in the regressing rat ventral prostate gland.

therefore the most stringent evidence we have obtained to date that prostate cell apoptosis and proliferation share the same early molecular pathway.

CONCLUSION

Androgenic steroids regulate the growth rate, differentiation state and lifespan of the prostate epithelial cell. Although each of these parameters would seem to be so different as to require completely different molecular mechanisms, we have obtained evidence that at least two of these pathways controlled by androgens – proliferation, and programmed death or apoptosis – occur through an identical early molecular pathway. Much of the evidence that we have obtained is based on showing that markers considered specific for proliferation (i.e. proto-oncogene and ODC expression, and tyrosine phosphorylation) are also induced in apoptotic prostate cells. Moreover, our BrdU incorporation studies functionally demonstrate that apoptotic prostate cells are also synthesizing DNA, thus corroborating the appearance of proliferation markers in the post-castrate ventral prostate gland.

Our results lead us to propose that the quiescent (G_0) prostate epithelial cells in a mature rat ventral prostate gland re-enter the cell cycle when androgenic steroids are removed. This is a very unexpected proposal since researchers have classically thought of androgenic steroids as the proliferative stimulus for prostate cells, whereas we are now suggesting that the abrupt removal of these steroids from prostate cells will also induce a cell cycle. This concept might be easier to understand when we better define the role that growth factors play in prostate cell biology. While we currently believe that androgen action alters the growth factor environment of the prostate gland in a manner conducive to a proliferative response, it is already clear that castration causes some abrupt changes in the expression of prostate growth factors that can affect cell behaviour. It is of note that renal tubular epithelial cell apoptosis induced by ureteral obstruction occurs in an environment modified by a rapid and drastic decline in the synthesis of epidermal growth factor in coordination with the increase in expression of renal transforming growth factor-β (Walton et al 1992). The most well characterized growth factor alteration in the post-castrate rat at this time is a rapid increase in the expression of transforming growth factor-β (Kyprianou & Isaacs 1989), and it is possible that this substance is a cofactor in prostate apoptosis, acting in conjunction with the loss of a required (yet undefined) prostatic growth factor. Further work in this area may help us to identify a growth factor environment that can predictably initiate prostate cell apoptosis.

If the differentiated prostate cells do re-enter the cell cycle after castration, it is clear that the cycle is never completed. Therefore we are also left to explain the defect in prostate cell cycle transition in the absence of testosterone. One area of increasing interest with regard to this question is a series of experiments demonstrating that activation of protein kinase-C can prevent cells from undergoing apoptosis (McConkey et al 1989, Perotti et al 1990). This enzyme is normally activated during a proliferation response. In preliminary experiments using an in vitro explant culture system with rat ventral prostate tissue, we have already found evidence that the phorbol ester, phorbol 12-myristate 13-acetate, a potent stimulator of protein kinase-C, can suppress apoptosis and the gene activity associated with this process in testosterone-free medium (Buttyan & Asase, preliminary communication). Thus, this potential defect – attempted proliferation with an inactive protein kinase-C – might be the common factor in many forms of apoptosis. Like the early growth factor environment of the regressing prostate gland, the proliferative machinery of the prostate cell will require further research to identify the site at which proliferation and apoptosis deviate.

In summary, apoptosis is a natural pathway that has evolved to eliminate cells from the body. To a great extent, we are fortunate that simple hormone manipulation can activate this death pathway in prostate cancer cells, efficiently providing a means for palliative relief of metastatic prostate cancer. However, since some prostate cancer cells are invariably resistant to hormonal therapy, there must be a block to this process in these insensitive prostate tumour cells that we hope, through our research, to identify and overcome. Rather than searching for simple lethal gene products, as was originally proposed as the cause of apoptosis, we now realize that, in many ways, this process is as complex as cellular proliferation. In fact, our evidence indicates that apoptosis is a process of defective proliferation. If we can identify this defect, we might be able to devise new strategies to enhance the effects of androgen deprivation and prolong survival of the metastatic prostate cancer patient.

REFERENCES

Bandyk M G, Sawczuk I S, Olsson C A et al 1990 Characterization of the products of a gene expressed during androgen-programmed cell death and their potential use as a marker of urogenetical injury. J Urol 143: 407–412

Batra S, Popper L D, Harley-Asp B 1991 Effect of calcium and calcium antagonists on ^{45}Ca influx and cellular growth of human prostatic tumor cells. Prostate 19: 299–307

Bruchovsky N, Lesser B, van Doorne E 1975 Hormonal effects on cell proliferation in the rat prostate. Vitam Horm 33: 61–102

Buttyan R 1991 Genetic response of prostate cells to androgen deprivation: Insights into the cellular mechanism of apoptosis. In: Tomei D, Cope F (eds) The Molecular Basis of Cell Death. Cold Spring Harbour Laboratory, New York, pp 157–173

Buttyan R, Zakeri Z, Locshin R et al 1988 Cascade induction of c-*fos*, c-*myc* and heat shock 70K transcripts during regression of the rat ventral prostate gland. Mol Endocrinol 2: 650–657

Chang C, Saltzman A G, Sorensen NS et al 1987 Identification of glutathione S-transferase Yb_1 mRNA as the androgen-repressed mRNA by cDNA cloning and sequence analysis. J Biol Chem 262: 11901–11903

Connor J, Sawczuk I S, Benson M C et al 1988 Calcium channel antagonists delay regression of androgen-dependent tissues and suppress gene activity associated with cell death. Prostate 13: 119–130

Di Fiore P P, Segatto O, Taylor W G et al 1990 EGF receptor and erbB-2 tyrosine kinase domains confer cell specificity for mitogenic signalling. Science 248: 79–83

Durham A C H, Walton J M 1982 Calcium ions and the control of proliferation in normal and cancer cells. Bioscience of Reproduction 2: 15–30

Ellis C, Moran M, McCormick et al 1990 Phosphorylation of GAP and GAP-associated proteins by transforming and mitogenic tyrosine kinases. Nature 343: 377–381

English H F, Kyprianou N, Isaacs J T 1989 Relationship between DNA fragmentation and apoptosis in the programmed cell death in the rat prostate following castration. Prostate 15: 233–250

Fantl W J, Escobedo J A, Williams L T 1989 Mutations of the platelet-derived growth factor receptor that cause a loss of ligand-induced conformational change, subtle changes in kinase activity, and impaired ability to stimulate DNA synthesis. Mol Cell Biol 9: 4473–4478

Hickok N J, Seppanen P J, Kontula K K et al 1986 Two ornithine decarboxylase mRNA species in mouse kidney arise from size heterogeneity at their 3′ termini. Proc Nat Acad Sci USA 83: 594–598

Katz A E, Benson M C, Wise G J et al 1989 Gene activity during the early phase of androgen-stimulated rat prostate regrowth. Cancer Res 49: 5889–5894

Kerr J R F, Searle J 1973 Deletion of cells by apoptosis during castration-induced involution of the rat prostate. Virchows Arch B Cell Pathol 13: 87–102

Kyprianou N, Isaacs J R 1989 Expression of transforming growth factor β in the rat ventral prostate during castration-induced programmed cell death. Mol Endocrinol 3: 1515–1522

Kyprianou N, English H F, Isaacs J T 1988 Activation of a Ca^{++}-Mg^{++}-dependent endonuclease as an early event in castration-induced prostate cell death. Prostate 13: 103–107

Laemmli U K 1970 Cleavage of structural proteins during the assembly of the head of bacteriophage T4. Nature 227: 680–682

Lee C 1981 Physiology of castration induced regression in the rat prostate. Prog Clin Biol Res 75: 145–159

McConkey D J, Hartzell P, Jondal M et al 1989 Inhibition of DNA fragmentation in thymocytes and isolated thymocyte nuclei by agents that stimulate protein kinase C. J Biol Chem 264: 13399–13402

Muller R, Bravo C, Burkhard I et al 1984 Induction of c-*fos* gene and protein by growth factors precedes the activation of c-*myc*. Nature 314: 546–548

Naldini L, Vigna E, Ferracini R et al 1991 The tyrosine kinase encoded by the *Met* proto-oncogene is activated by autophosphorylation. Mol Cell Biol 11: 1793–1803

Perotti M, Toddei F, Mirabelli et al 1990 Federation of the Society for Experimental Biology Letters 259: 331–334

Rolink A, Streb M, Nishikawa et al 1991 The c-kit-encoded tyrosine kinase regulates the proliferation of early pre-B cells. Eur J Immunol 21: 2609–2612

Sanford M L, Searle J W, Kerr J F R 1984 Successive waves of apoptosis in the rat prostate after repeated withdrawal of testosterone stimulation. Pathology 16: 406–410

Schutte B, Reynders M M J, Bosman F T et al 1987 Studies with anti-bromodeoxyuridine antibodies: II. Simultaneous immunocytochemical detection of antigen expression and DNA synthesis by in vivo labelling of mouse intestinal mucosa. J Histochem Cytochem 35: 371–374

Sensibar J A, Liu X, Patai B et al 1990 Characterization of castration-induced cell death in the rat prostate by immunohistochemical localization of cathepsin D. Prostate 16: 263–276

Stanisic T R, Sadlowsky R, Lee C et al 1978 Partial inhibition of castration induced ventral prostate regression with actinomycin D and cyclohexamide. Invest Urol 16: 19–22

Thompson N L, Mead J E, Braun L et al 1986 Sequential protooncogene expression during rat liver regeneration. Cancer Res 46: 3111–3117

Williams-Ashman H G, Canellakis Z N 1979 Polyamines in mammalian biology and medicine. Perspect Biol Med 22: 421–453

Walton G, Buttyan R, Garcia-Montes E et al 1992 Renal growth factor expression during the early phase of experimental hydronephrosis. J Urol in press

Yoneda T, Lyall R M, Alsina M M et al 1991 The antiproliferative effects of tyrosine kinase inhibitors tyrosphostins on a human squamous cell carcinoma in vitro and in nude mice. Cancer Res 51: 4430–4435

17. Correlation between restriction fragment length polymorphism of the L-myc gene and lymph node metastasis in prostate cancer

G. E. Chechile   E. A. Klein   R. Connelly   H. Levin

INTRODUCTION

The myc family of cellular proto-oncogenes consists of three members: c-myc, N-myc and L-myc and are known to be involved in a variety of different cancers. L-myc was first identified in human small cell lung cancer (SCLC) by its limited homology to both c-myc and N-myc. Restriction endonuclease EcoRI digests of human DNA produce a fragment length polymorphism of L-myc defined by two alleles, a 10.0-kilobase (kb) 'L' and a 6.6-kb 'S' allele (Nau et al 1985).

Kato et al (1990) have shown that patients homozygous or heterozygous for the S allele (SS or SL) of L-myc have an increased risk of bone and soft tissue sarcoma development. Kakehi & Hoshida (1989) and Kawashima et al (1988) found a correlation between increased metastasis and the S allele of L-myc in patients with renal and SCLC patients, respectively. Saranath et al (1990) reported that oral cancer patients with a genotype including an S fragment are more likely to develop a larger or a poor differentiated tumour than are patients without an S fragment.

We have analyzed a group of patients with clinically localized adenocarcinoma of the prostate to determine if the pattern of L and S alleles could serve as a marker for biologically aggressive prostatic tumours.

MATERIALS AND METHODS

Patients

We studied 37 patients with clinically localized prostatic cancer who underwent bilateral pelvic lymphadenectomy and radical prostatectomy with curative intent. In all patients, cancer was histologically certified via needle or aspiration biopsy prior to surgery. Metastatic disease was ruled out by standard clinical staging.

Tumour samples

A pathologist guided by preoperative localization studies and digital palpation obtained several cores of tumour with an 18-gauge tru-cut needle. The presence of cancer was immediately confirmed by frozen section. Normal prostatic tissue was similarly obtained and verified. Tumour and normal samples were frozen in liquid nitrogen immediately after surgery and stored. A blood sample was also obtained from each patient.

DNA isolation, probe labelling and Southern blot analysis

High-molecular-weight DNA was extracted from tumour, normal prostate and white blood cells by conventional methods. Ten μg of DNA per sample were digested with EcoRI, separated by 0.8% agarose gel electrophoresis and transferred to nitrocellulose filter by standard blotting procedures (Southern 1975).

The L-myc probe, a 1.8-kb SmaI-EcoRI fragment cloned in pJB327, was obtained from O. Yoshida (Kyoto University) via the Japanese Cancer Research Resource Bank. The filters were hybridized with the L-myc probe labelled with ^{32}P by random oligonucleotide primer technique (Feinberg & Vogelstein 1983). The filters were then washed in 0.1 × SSC and 0.1 SDS and exposed to Kodak XAR film at −70°C.

Histopathology

Pelvic lymph nodes were formalin-fixed, sectioned and stained with haematoxylin and eosin (H&E) for histological analysis. Whole prostates were formalin-fixed for 72 hours, inked with two colours, step-sectioned from the apex to the seminal vesicles at 5-mm intervals and stained with H&E. All tumours were TMN classified according to the UICC guidelines (1989). The Gleason system was used for grade classification.

RESULTS

Of the 37 patients, six had microscopic nodal metastasis in one or two lymph nodes as well as seminal vesicle invasion (P3bN1M0). Of the 31 patients without pelvic node invasion, four had cancers confined to the prostate (P2N0M0), 19 had capsular invasion or penetration (P3aN0M0) and 14 had seminal vesicle involvement (P3bN0M0).

The grade was moderately differentiated in 14 patients and poorly differentiated in 23 patients.

Nine patients were genetically homozygous for the 10-kb L-myc fragment (LL), 10 were homozygous for the 6.6-kb fragment (SS), and 18 were heterozygous (LS). The relationship between L-myc restriction fragment length polymorphism and the presence or absence of nodal involvement is shown in Table 17.1.

Table 17.1 Correlation of L-myc alleles and the incidence of lymph node metastasis.

	Allelic pattern			Allelic frequency	
	LL	LS	SS	L	S
Total cases	9	18	10		
N+	0	3	3	0.250	0.750
N−	9	15	7	0.532	0.468

N+ = nodal involvement N− = no nodal involvement

Table 17.2 Relationship between L-myc alleles and seminal vesicle invasion

	Allelic pattern			Allelic frequency	
	LL	LS	SS	L	S
Total cases	9	18	10		
Invasion +	1	8	5	0.357	0.643
Invasion −	8	10	5	0.565	0.435

Of the six patients who exhibited nodal metastases, all represented either the LS or SS type polymorphic pattern; no patient homozygous for the L allele (LL) had positive nodes.

The distribution of the L-myc allele as a function of seminal vesicle invasion showed a trend toward more S alleles in patients with invasion (Table 17.2). Fourteen patients (38%) presented seminal vesicle invasion and 13 showed the S fragment in the genotype; only one patient was homozygous for the L allele. There was no significant correlation between presence or absence of S fragment and either grade or stage of the tumours (Table 17.3).

Table 17.3 Relationship between L-myc alleles and histopathological stage

	Allelic pattern			Allelic frequency	
Stage	LL	LS	SS	L	S
P2N0M0	1	3	0	0.625	0.375
P3aN0M0	7	7	5	0.553	0.447
P3bN0M0	1	8	5	0.357	0.643
Total cases	9	18	10		

DISCUSSION

This study was conducted to investigate whether we could confirm the correlation between the presence of the S allele of L-myc and an increased incidence of metastasis to lymph nodes in patients with clinically localized prostate cancer undergoing radical prostatectomy.

The overall frequencies of alleles (L= 0.49 and S= 0.51) observed in the study population were similar to those reported in the general population, suggesting that the risk of developing prostate cancer is not affected by the L-myc allelic pattern.

Of our 37 patients, six (16%) exhibited pelvic node metastases. Surprisingly, none of the six patients showed the LL genotype. These findings are consistent with the results observed in patients with renal cancer (Kakehi & Yoshida 1989) and lung cancer (Kawashima et al 1988).

On the other hand, Tefre et al (1990) and Ikede et al (1988) failed to demonstrate a correlation between the L-myc genotype SS and increased metastasis to lymph nodes and distal organs in patients with lung and colorectal cancer, respectively. According to Tefre et al (1990) there are three possible explanations for this discrepancy:

a. random variation, which tends to occur when the populations studied are small
b. stratification in the ascertainment of the patients
c. linkage desequilibrium.

We also found a trend toward more S alleles in patients with invasion of the seminal vesicles. However, we found no difference in the distribution of the alleles as a function of capsular confinement or invasion, clinical stage or grade, previous radiation or hormonal therapy or the presence of tumour at the surgical margin of the specimen.

The results of our study suggest that L-myc restriction fragment length polymorphism may serve as a useful genetic market for biologically aggressive prostatic tumours.

REFERENCES

Feinberg A P, Vogelstein B 1983 A technique for radiolabeling DNA restriction endonuclease fragments to high specific activity. Ann Biochem 132: 6–13

Ikeda I, Ishizaka Y, Ochiai M et al 1988 No correlation between L-myc restriction fragment length polymorphism and malignancy of human colorectal cancers. Jpn J Cancer Res 79: 674–676

Nau M M, Brooks B J, Battley J et al 1985 L-myc, a new myc related gene amplified and expressed in human small cell lung cancer. Nature 318: 69–73

Kakehi Y, Yoshida O 1989 Restriction fragment length polymorphism of the L-myc gene and susceptibility to metastasis in renal cancer patients. Int J Cancer 43: 391–394

Kato M, Toguchida J, Honda K et al 1990 Elevated frequency of a specific allele of the L-myc gene in male patients with bone and soft-tissue sarcomas. Int J Cancer 45: 47–49

Kawashima A, Shikama H, Imoto K et al 1988 Close correlation between restriction fragment length polymorphism of the L-myc gene and metastasis of human lung cancer to the lymph nodes and other organs. Proc Nat Acad Sci USA 85: 2353–2356

Saranath D, Panchal R G, Nair R et al 1990 Restriction fragment length polymorphism of the L-myc gene in oral cancer patients. Br J Cancer 61: 530–533

Southern E M 1975 Detection of specific sequences among DNA fragments separated by gel electrophoresis. J Mol Biol 98: 503–517

Tefre T, Borresen A L, Aamdal S et al 1990 Studies of the L-myc DNA polymorphism and relation to metastasis in norwegian lung cancer patients. Br J Cancer 61: 809–812

18. Alterations of the p53 gene are involved in the progression of a human prostate carcinoma

P. J. Effert A. Neubauer P. J. Walther E. T. Liu

INTRODUCTION

Correlates of molecular genetic alterations with clinical disease progression have been an increasing focus of attention in the study of human prostate carcinoma. Increased DNA content, when determined by flow cytometry, can predict an adverse treatment outcome, even in localized disease (Lee et al 1988). However, in contrast to other tumour systems, little is known about specific genetic alterations relevant to prostate carcinogenesis. A Ki-ras mutation was observed in a prostatic adenocarcinoma (Peehl et al 1987); and an activated Ha-ras oncogene was seen in 1/24 prostate cancer specimens (Carter et al 1990a).

The importance of another class of genes, commonly referred to as tumour suppressor genes (or 'anti-oncogenes'), becomes increasingly evident from studies of other tumours. In clinical prostate cancer, however, little evidence exists for alterations in these genes. Observations of chromosomal deletions have been noted (Atkin et al 1985, Carter et al 1990b) that suggest the possibility of loss of critical genes (potentially suppressor genes). Bookstein et al (1990) recently identified a mutation in the promoter region of one in seven primary prostate tumours, suggesting that specific tumour suppressor genes are involved in prostate carcinogenesis.

The p53 gene is a tumour suppressor gene which has been implicated in the molecular genetics of several common human malignancies. Nucleotide alterations, most commonly single point mutations, have been shown to not only abrogate the p53 suppressor function but also contribute to the transformed phenotype. Among others, p53 mutations have been identified in breast, colon, lung and bladder carcinomas. Also consistent with the hypothesis of p53 as a tumour suppressor gene is the finding of frequent loss of genes on chromosomes 17p in many common adult tumours such as those of the colon, breast, lung and bladder.

To date, p53 mutations have not yet been reported in clinical prostate cancer. Also, little or no work defining the nature of p53 genetic alterations in primary clinical specimens versus corresponding metastases has been performed. We were presented with the opportunity to analyze tumour material retrieved from a primary prostate adenocarcinoma as well as its deposit in a regional lymph node. We report the detection of a point mutation in an evolutionary conserved region in the fifty exon of the p53 gene. The heterogeneity of this somatic mutation in the primary specimen and the additional loss of heterozygosity on chromosome 17p in the metastasis would suggest that these events may participate in the progression of human prostate cancer.

MATERIAL AND METHODS

Case report

Tumour specimens were retrieved from primary prostate cancer and a regional lymph node metastasis of the same tumour in a 67-year-old male who underwent radical cystoprostatectomy for locally advanced prostate cancer. The patient had received external beam teletherapy (6500 rads) 14 years earlier when prostate cancer was first diagnosed.

Pathology

On histopathologic examination, diffuse infiltration of the prostate gland was noted. A Gleason pattern of 4/3 was noted. At the sites where tissue was removed for genetic analysis, tumour area determination showed 91% of the area to be involved. One of the regional lymph nodes was completely replaced by undifferentiated tumour (100% by tumour area analysis), a portion of which was immediately preserved for subsequent analysis.

Genetic analytic methodology

Tissues were processed at the time of surgery. DNA was extracted from snap-frozen tissues and peripheral blood cells of the patient using standard methodology (Maniatis 1982). For histopathologic assessment, tissues were formalin-fixed and paraffin-embedded.

A 2.9-kb fragment of p53, containing exons 4–9, was preamplified, and amplified fragments were isolated from a preparative 1% agarose gel. These purified fragments were used as a template for subsequent SSCP-analysis (Orita et al 1989), which allows for screening of a point mutation in exons 5, 7 and 8 of the p53 gene by assessing abnormal electrophoretic mobility of polymerase chain reaction (PCR)-amplified DNA sequences labelled with incorporated ^{32}P-dCTP.

The 29-kb preamplified fragments were also used for direct DNA-sequencing and subjected to a second asymmetric PCR-reaction (Dicker et al 1989) using different primer pairs for exons 5, 7 and 8. The concentration of primers was 0.5 μM and 0.01 μM, respectively. Both strands were subsequently sequenced by the modification of Sanger's method using the respective primers in the sequencing reactions.

Detection of allelic loss

Probe YNZ 22 detects a highly polymorphic VNTR segment on chromosome 17p (Nakamura et al 1987). Primers directing amplification across the YNZ 22 region were recently described (Horn et al 1989). Amplification was performed under standard conditions with 1 µg of genomic DNA. One tenth of the amplification products was electrophoresed on 8% polyacrylamide gels and visualized by ethidium bromide staining.

RESULTS AND DISCUSSION

After standardizing the conditions, SSCP analysis proved to be a rapid and sensitive screening tool for the detection of point mutations in the p53 gene. Analyses were performed on tissues corresponding exactly to areas containing mainly tumour cells. When amplified fragments of exon 5 were subjected to SSCP-analysis, abnormal electrophoretic mobility was reproducibly noted in different DNA samples of the lymph node metastasis. Of two DNA samples obtained from the primary tumour tissue, however, only one displayed such abnormal electrophoretic migration. These results, indicating the presence of point mutations in part of the primary and all the metastatic tumour tissue, could subsequently be confirmed by direct DNA-sequencing. A mutation (GTT to GCT) at codon 172, substituting valine by alanine in the p53 protein sequence, was identified in part of the primary and all the metastatic tissue. This indicates that the primary tumour was composed of a heterogenous population of tumour cells: one area being populated by tumour cells harbouring a mutant p53-allele and other areas containing cells without p53 mutations. The location of the mutation identified is in agreement with data obtained in other tumour systems; many mutations have been mapped to highly conserved sequences in exons 5, 7 and 8 (Nigro et al 1989).

Though the p53 mutations may mark cells that later acquire metastatic behaviour, perturbation of p53 alone did not appear to have induced the metastasis since the same mutation was detected in both primary and metastatic tumour cells. When DNA samples from peripheral blood cells and primary and metastatic tumour tissue were subsequently analyzed for somatic allelic loss of chromosome 17p sequence, two alleles were found in blood cells and primary tumour. In the metastasis, however, allelic loss on the short arm of chromosome 17p was detected. Since this allelic loss did involve the p53 gene itself, it appears possible that a gene different from p53 but linked to YNZ 22 locus was lost in the metastatic process. This is also supported by recent findings implicating a gene other than p53 on the short arm of chromosome 17p in human breast carcinogenesis (Coles et al 1990, Chen et al 1991).

In conclusion, this study has identified two genetic alterations in a human prostate carcinoma, that appear to be associated with clinical tumour progression. The determination of the prevalence of these alterations as well as the association of these parameters with grade and stage of prostatic adenocarcinomas might point to valuable indicators for stratification of disease outcome.

REFERENCES

Atkin N B, Baker M C 1985 Chromosome study of five cancers of the prostate. Hum Genet 70: 359–364

Carter B S, Epstein J I, Isaacs W B 1990 Ras gene mutations in human prostate cancer. Cancer Res 50: 6830–6832

Carter B S, Ewing C M, Ward W S et al 1990b Allelic loss of chromosomes 16q and 10q in human prostate cancer. Proc Nat Acad Sci USA 87: 8751–8755

Chen L-C, Neubauer A, Kurisu W 1991 A gene other than p53 on the short arm of chromosome 17 is associated with high proliferative capacity and DNA aneuploidy in primary human breast cancer. Proc Nat Acad Sci USA (in press)

Coles C, Thompson A M, Elder P A 1990 Evidence implicating at least two genes on chromosome 17p in breast carcinogenesis. Lancet 336: 761–3

Dicker A P, Volkenandt M, Adamo 1939 Sequence analysis of a human gene: A rapid method for manual and automated direct sequencing of products generated by the polymerase chain reaction. Biotechniques 7: 830–838

Horn G T, Richards B, Klinger K W 1989 Amplification of a highly polymorphic VNTR segment by the polymerase chain reaction. Nucleic Acids Res 17: 2140

Lee S E, Currin S M, Paulson D F 1988 Flow cytometric determination of ploidy in prostate adenocarcinoma: a comparison with seminal vesicle involvement and histopathologic grading as predictors of clinical recurrence. J Urol 140: 769–774

Maniatis T, Fritsch E F, Sambrook J 1982 Molecular cloning: a laboratory manual. Cold Spring Harbor Laboratory Press, New York

Nakamura Y, Leppert M, O'Connell P 1987 Variable number of tandem repeat markers for human gene mapping. Science 235: 1616–1622

Nigro J M, Baker S J, Preisinger A C 1939 Mutations in the p53 gene occur in diverse human tumour types. Nature 342: 705–708

Orita M, Suzuki Y, Sekiya T 1989 Rapid and sensitive detection of point mutations and DNA polymorphisms using the polymerase chain reaction. Genomics 5: 874–879

Peehl D M, Wehner N, Stamey T A 1987 Activated c-Ki-ras proto-oncogene in human prostatic adenocarcinoma. Prostate 10: 281–287

19. Progression of androgen-dependent tumour to androgen-independent tumour

Y. Furuya   N. Sato   Y. Watabe   J. Shimazaki

SUMMARY

An autonomous subline (CS 2) derived from androgen-dependent Shionogi Carcinoma 115 (SC 115) expressed hst-1 gene, which was not expressed in SC 115. Transfection of the hst-1 gene into SC 115 evoked the malignant phenotype with partial loss of androgen dependency. The hst-1 gene was therefore suggested to play some role in the progression of androgen-dependent tumours.

CS 2 secreted fibroblast-growth-factor-like growth factor which controlled the growth of CS 2 and the parent SC 115 in autocrine and paracrine manners, respectively, although the relationship between hst-1 expression and production of the growth factor was not clarified. Suramin inhibited the activity of this factor by blocking the binding with its cell surface receptor. These results indicated that progression to the autonomous tumour requires new phenotypes including expression of the oncogene and secretion of the growth factor.

Approximately 80% of advanced prostatic cancer patients respond to endocrine therapy at the start of treatment, but more than half of the responders gradually lose responsiveness (Catalona & Scott 1978). This progression to hormone-resistant disease during hormonal therapy is thus one of the most serious problems in prostatic cancer. To clarify the progression further, we have been working with androgen-dependent mouse tumour (Shionogi Carcinoma 115, SC 115). Using SC 115 and its autonomous subline, it was shown that oncogene expression and growth factor secretion played an important role in the progression of SC 115.

TUMOURS

SC 115 was established in 1964 as an androgen-dependent tumour (Minesita & Yamaguchi 1964). Chiba Subline 2 (CS 2) is an androgen-independent subline derived from SC 115 (Fuse et al 1983). Both SC 115 and CS 2 contain the androgen receptor. Modal chromosomal numbers of SC 115 and CS 2 are 40 and 72, respectively (Zama et al 1987), but these tumours share common marker chromosomes, indicating that CS 2 ori-

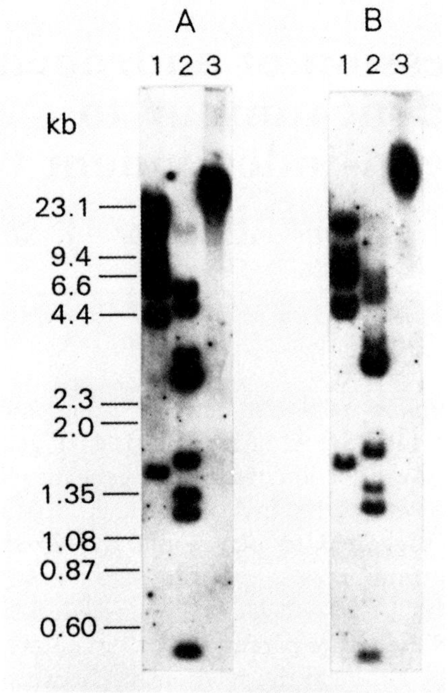

Fig. 19.1 Southern blot analysis of genomic DNA from SC 115 (**A**) and CS 2 (**B**) cells. Genomic DNA was extracted, digested with EcoRI (lane 1) or MspI (lane 2), or not digested (lane 3). Hybridization was performed with a probe of MMTV-LTR. HindIII digest of λDNA and HaeIII digest of φX174 were used as markers. (Reprinted from Akakura et al 1990)

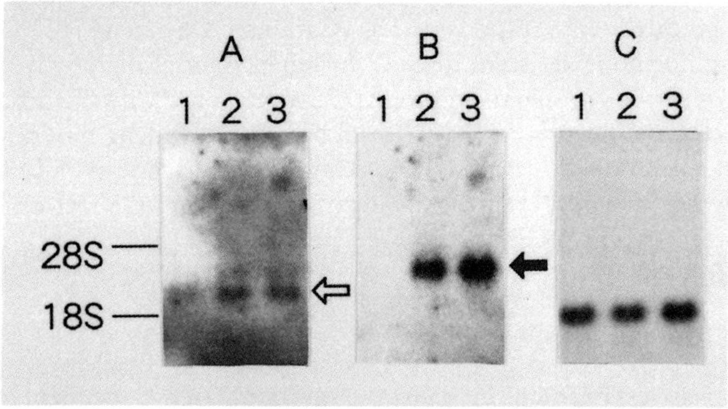

Fig. 19.2 Northern blot analysis of RNA obtained after culturing SC 115 or CS 2 in the presence (lane 1: SC 115, lane 2: CS 2) or absence (lane 3: CS 2) of 10^{-8}M testosterone. For electrophoresis, 3 μ of poly(A)$^+$ RNA/lane was applied. Hybridization was performed with probes of int–2 (**A**), hst-1 (**B**) and β-actin (**C**). Arrows indicate the positions of transcripts of int–2 (2.7 kb) and hst-1 (3.2 kb). Positions of ribosomal RNA are indicated. (Reprinted from Akakura et al 1990)

ginated from SC 115. SC 115 and CS 2 cells have been cloned with retention of the respective androgen responsiveness and unresponsiveness (Furuya et al 1990a,b). These cell lines were used throughout the work.

EXPRESSION OF hst-1

The hst-1 gene was first identified by transfection of NIH/3T3 cells with human DNA samples obtained from a gastric cancer (Sakamoto et al 1986). Sequencing analysis of a murine homologue of the hst-1 gene revealed that it encoded a protein of 202 amino acids which had 82% homology to human hst-1 (Brookes et al 1989). It was reported that mouse mammary tumour virus (MMTV) evoked the expression of int-2 and hst-1 (Peters et al 1989), and the integration of MMTV was also detected in the SC 115 (Darbre et al 1983). Therefore, the integration of MMTV and oncogene expressions in SC 115 and CS 2 cells were compared. Restriction fragments hybridized with long terminal repeat (LTR) of MMTV showed almost identical patterns between SC 115 and CS 2 cells after digestion with EcoRI and MspI (Fig. 19.1), and the patterns were similar to those reported by Darbre et al (1983). The new insertion of MMTV was not found in CS 2. Weak expression of the int-2 gene was observed in the two cells, but expression of the hst-1 gene was seen only in CS 2 (Fig. 19.2). In Southern blot analysis, restriction fragments digested with BamHI in CS 2 showed an additional short fragment when compared with those in SC 115. This may be explained by some DNA rearrangements near the hst-1 gene locus in CS 2, and these changes might evoke the expression of hst-1. Consequently, the expression of hst-1 seems to be related to the autonomous growth of CS 2.

TRANSFECTION OF hst-1

To clarify the significance of hst-1 expression, hst-1 expression vector was introduced into SC 115 cells, and the characteristics of transfectants were investigated. Transfection of DNA into SC 115 cells was performed according to the method of calcium phosphate precipitation with the plasmids pKOneo, pKOc5, and pZB5. pKOc5 and pZB5 possess the hst-1 gene, driven by SV40 early promoter and murine leukaemia virus LTR, respectively (Taira et al 1987). The transfectant with pKOneo, which possessed the bacterial neomycin-resistance gene, was used as a control. After transfection, cells were exposed to a media containing 500 μg/ml of the antibiotics G418, and G418-resistant colonies were isolated, designated as SC115/neo, SC115/c5 and SC115/ZB5, and used for the study. SC 115 and SC115/neo cells grew exponentially in the presence of 10^{-8} M testosterone, and the growth rate of 115/neo was almost identical to that of SC 115 cells (Fig. 19.3). In the absence of testosterone, these two cells did not proliferate, showing androgen dependency. The growth rates of SC 115/c5 and SC 115/ZB5 in the presence of testosterone were significantly higher

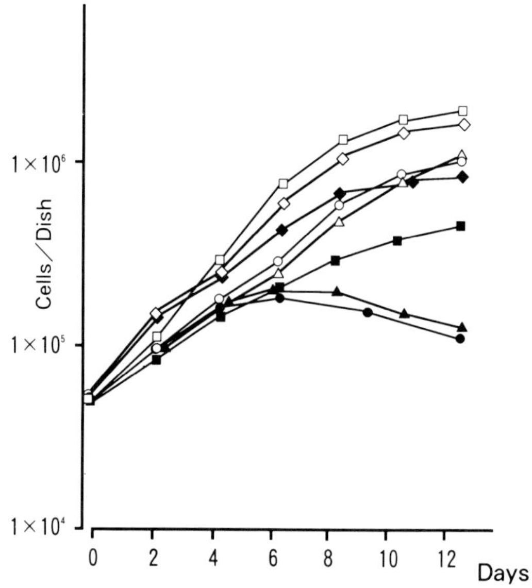

Fig. 19.3 Growth of SC 115 cells and transfectants of hst-1 and/or neomycin resistance genes. Cells were cultured in MEM/Ham's F-12 containing 1% FBS with (open symbols) or without (closed symbols) 10^{-8}M testosterone. SC 115 (triangle), SC 115/neo (circle), SC 115/c5 (diamond) and SC 115/ZB5 (square). (Reprinted from Furuya et al 1991.)

than those of SC115 and SC 115/neo cells. These two cells showed growth even in the absence of testosterone, although the growth rate was lower than that in the presence of testosterone.

SC 115 and SC115/neo cells did not form colonies in soft agar without testosterone. However, approximately 10 colonies/dish appeared in the cultures of SC 115 and SC 115/neo in the presence of testosterone (Table 19.1). SC 115/c5 and SC 115/ZB5 formed colonies in the absence of testosterone, but the effect of testosterone on colony formation was evident.

Table 19.1 Anchorage-independent growth of SC 115 cells and transfectants of hst-1 and/or neomycin-resistant genes

Cell line	Colonies/dish* With testosterone	Without testosterone
SC 115	0	8 ± 2
SC 115/neo	0	6 ± 1
SC 115/c5	24 ± 5	174 ± 15
SC 115/ZB5	28 ± 5	60 ± 10

*The cells were cultured in soft agar with or without 10^{-8} M testosterone.
(Modified from Furuya et al 1991.)

SC 115 and SC115/neo cells showed a fibroblast-like shape in the presence of androgen, but removal of testosterone changed the shape to epithelial-like morphology by phase contrast microscopy. SC 115/c5 and SC 115/ZB5 showed a fibroblast-like appearance regardless of the presence or absence of testosterone. The latter two formed distinct foci in which the cells were piled up.

After transplantation of SC 115 and SC 115/neo cells in male mice of the DD/S strain, small nodules less than 0.5 cm in diameter appeared in a few animals, but further growth of nodules did not occur during 12 weeks. However, SC 115/c5 and 115/ZB5 cells formed tumours in male DD/S mice, although there was little tumour formation in female ones. The tumour which arose after inoculation of SC 115/c5 and SC 115/ZB5 cells showed poorly differentiated adenocarcinoma, which resembled the original SC 115. Metastatic foci did not appear in mice bearing SC 115/c5 and SC 115/ZB5 cells up to 12 weeks of the experimental period.

From the transfection experiments, it was concluded that the transfectants with the hst-1 gene preserved androgen-responsiveness in their growth, but they might acquire malignant potential when compared with parent SC 115 cells. Acquired malignant potential in the transfectant seems to be related to the expression of hst-1, since control transfectants with pKOneo showed no new characteristics as compared with SC 115 cells.

SECRETION OF GROWTH FACTOR FROM CS 2

It has been reported that the growth of SC 115 cells required androgen in serum-free medium (Nonomura et al 1988). CS 2 cells grew equally when in the presence or absence of androgen in serum-free conditions. When two cells were cultured together in the ratio 1:1, both cells grew equally well irrespective of the presence or absence of testosterone (Fig. 19.4). This suggested that CS 2 cells supported the growth of SC 115 cells even without androgen. To define this growth-stimulating effect, conditioned medium from serum-free cultures of CS 2 cells was prepared, and the growth-promoting activity in the conditioned medium was examined. The medium stimulated thymidine incorporation into the DNA of both SC 115 cells and CS 2 cells in a dose-independent manner, showing that growth factor(s) secreted from CS 2 cells promoted cell growth in autocrine and paracrine manners. Therefore, the activity was measured by thymidine uptake into SC 115 cells.

Since the factor revealed affinity to heparin, conditioned medium obtained from CS 2 cells was purified using heparin affinity chromatography. After two cycles of heparin affinity chromatography followed by size exclusion chromatography, the factor showed a molecular weight of approximately 50000, which was confirmed with sodium dodecyl sulphate-polyacrylamide gel electrophoresis. The factor was relatively resistant to heat treatment but trypsin treatment completely abolished the

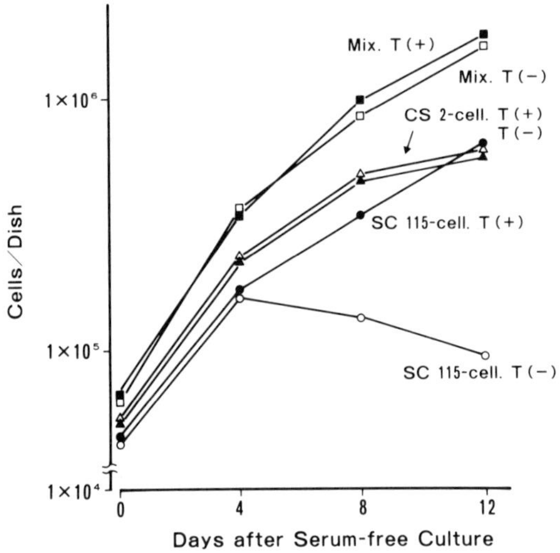

Fig. 19.4 Growth of SC 115 and CS 2 cells cultured separately or in combination (Mix.). Cells were cultured in 10% FBS-containing medium for two days and transferred to the serum-free medium with [T(+)] or without [T(−)] 10^{-8}M testosterone. In mixed culture, the ratio of SC 115 and CS 2 cells was 1:1 at the start of culture. (Reprinted from Furuya et al 1990a.)

activity. Among known growth factors – including fibroblast growth factors (FGF), epidermal growth factor, transforming growth factors and insulin-like growth factors – only acidic and basic FGFs had growth-promoting

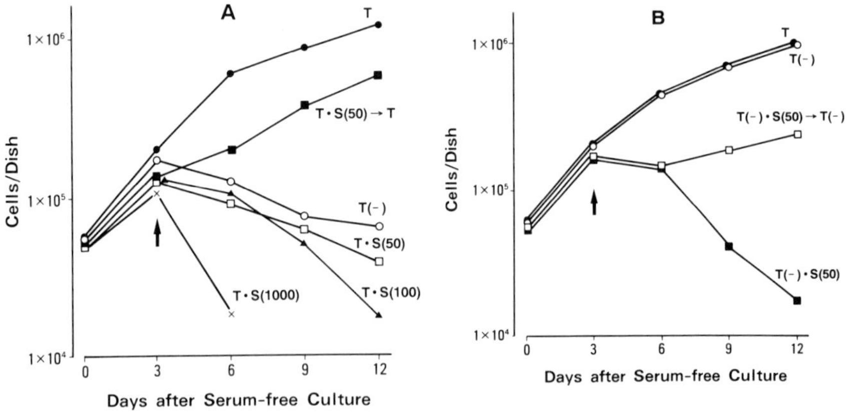

Fig. 19.5 Effects of suramin on growth of SC 115 (**A**) and CS 2 (**B**) cells. SC 115 and CS 2 cells were cultured with [T] or without [T(−)] 10^{-8}M testosterone. Suramin was supplemented at concentrations of 50 [S(50)], 100 [S(100)], or 1000 [S(1000)] µg/ml. In some dishes, suramin was removed from the culture medium at the times indicated (arrows). (Reprinted from Furuya et al 1990b.)

effects on SC 115 cells. Anti-basic-FGF antibody partially blocked the activity of growth factor secreted from CS 2 cells.

It was reported that using serum-free culture, the growth of SC 115 was regulated by an FGF-like peptide which was synthesized in the presence of androgen (Nonomura et al 1988). In this study, the CS 2 cell, an autonomous subline of SC 115, was shown to produce the growth factor which possessed properties similar to those of FGF. These two FGF-like peptides share common properties – an affinity to heparin, stability to heat and acid treatments, decreased activity in the presence of anti-basic FGF antibody – but differ in other respects, i.e. molecular weight, etc.

CS 2 cells also appear to have less necrotic tendency when compared with SC 115 (Ichikawa et al 1989), and the FGF-like peptide produced by CS 2 cells may contribute to prevention of the necrotic process. CS 2 cells express the hst-1 gene (see above), but further studies are required to determine whether the growth factor secreted from CS 2 cells is the hst-1 product or not. Addition of suramin inhibited the growth of SC 115 and CS 2 cells in a dose-dependent manner (Fig. 19.5). Suramin inhibits the growth-promoting activity of the growth factor secreted by CS 2 cells, by blocking its binding to the cell surface receptor. Our results indicate that suramin may be useful as an anti-cancer drug for both androgen-dependent and androgen-independent tumours.

REFERENCES

Akakura K, Furuya Y, Sato N et al 1990 Acquired expression of *hst–1* in a autonomous subline (Chiba Subline 2) derived from androgen-responsive mouse mammary tumour (Shionogi Carcinoma 115). Jpn Cancer Res 81: 554–556

Brookes S, Smith R, Thurlow J et al 1989 The mouse homologue of hst/k-FGF: sequence, genome organization and location relative to int-2. Nucleic Acids Res 17: 4037–4045

Catalona W J, Scott W W 1978 Carcinoma of the prostate. J Urol 119: 1–8

Darbre P, Dickson C, Peters G et al 1983 Androgen regulation of cell proliferation and expression of viral sequences in mouse mammary tumor cells. Nature 303: 431–433

Furuya Y, Sato N, Akakura K 1990a Paracrine growth stimulation of androgen-responsive Shionogi Carcinoma 115 by its autonomous subline (Chiba Subline 2). Cancer Res 50: 4979–4983

Furuya Y, Sato N, Watabe Y et al 1990b Effect of suramin on growth of androgen-responsive mouse tumor (Shionogi Carcinoma 115) and its autonomous subline (Chiba Subline 2). Endocrinol Jpn 37: 933–942

Furuya Y, Sato N, Watabe Y et al 1991 Appearance of malignant phenotype with partial loss of hormone dependency in androgen-dependent Shionogi Carcinoma 115 transfected with *hst–1* gene. Jpn J Cancer Res 82, in press

Fuse H, Akimoto S, Sato R et al 1983 Changes in cytosolic androgen receptor after administration of testosterone of androgen-dependent mouse mammary tumor (Shionogi Carcinoma) and its sublines of altered androgen dependency. Endocrinol Jpn 30: 189–197

Ichikawa T, Akimoto S, Hayata I et al 1989 Progression and selection in heterogeneous tumor composed of androgen-responsive Shionogi Carcinoma 115 and its autonomous subline (Chiba Subline 2). Cancer Res 49: 367–371

Minesita T, Yamaguchi K 1964 An androgen-dependent tumor of a female mouse. Steroids 4: 815–830

Nonomura N, Nakamura N, Uchida N 1988 Growth-stimulatory effect of androgen-induced autocrine growth factor(s) secreted from Shionogi Carcinoma 115 cells on androgen-unresponsive cancer cells in a paracrine mechanism. Cancer Res 48: 4904–4908

Peters G, Brookes S, Smith R et al 1989 The mouse homolog of the hst/k-FGF gene is adjacent to int-2 and is activated by proviral insertion in some virally induced mammary tumors. Proc Natl Acad Sci USA 86: 5678–5682

Sakamoto H, Mori M, Taira M et al 1986 Transforming gene from human stomach cancers and a noncancerous portion of stomach mucosa. Proc Natl Acad Sci USA 83: 3997–4001

Taira M, Yoshida T, Miyagawa K et al 1987 cDNA sequence of human transforming gene hst and identification of the coding sequence required for transforming activity. Proc Natl Acad Sci USA 84: 2980–2984

Zama S, Akimoto S, Yazawa S et al 1987 Androgen receptor testosterone uptake and karyotype in androgen-dependent mouse tumor (SC 115) and its androgen-independent subline (CS 2). Endocrinol Jpn 34: 279–289

20. Allelotype of urothelial and prostatic cancers

K. Kazuto V. P. Collins U. S. R. Bergerheim
L. Andersson J. H. Hisazumi

INTRODUCTION

Genotype analysis has considerably extended our understanding of the pathogenesis of cancer (Cossman 1990). One line of evidence has demonstrated that human cancers of diverse types arise through the combined genetic events of oncogene activations and the inactivation of tumour suppressor genes (TSGs) in the genome. While the oncogene family has mainly been identified in cancer-inducing retroviruses, TSGs have been shown to be inactivated in vivo in the human cancer genome although the original concept of TSG was deduced from cell fusion experiments (Harris et al 1969).

A series of studies in both hereditary and sporadic forms of retinoblastomas have indicated that a TSG, the Retinoblastoma 1 (Rb1) gene is activated in retinoblastoma cells, thus suggesting a critical role in oncogenesis (Knudson 1971, 1976, Benedict et al 1983, Cavenee et al 1983, Cavenee & Hansen 1988). In this series, restriction fragment length polymorphism (RFLP) analysis of paired normal and tumour DNA from the same patient revealed that loss of certain chromosomal regions of the tumour genome implied the fact that certain TSG(s) was inactivated in the regions, which was demonstrated afterward by some investigators (Friend et al 1986, 1987, Huang et al 1988, Bookstein et al 1989). RFLP analysis has been applied to a variety of human cancers to search for the involvement of inactivated TSGs in each tumour type (Green 1988, Sager 1989). At present, for example, the p53 gene on the short arm of chromosome 17 (17p) and DCC genes on the long arm of chromosome 18 (18q) are recorded as a TSG family (Nigro et al 1989, Sidransky et al 1991, Fearon et al 1990).

STRATEGIES OF RFLP ANALYSIS

RFLP

Although each cell has two copies of every chromosome, the DNA sequence of homologous chromosomes differs in a single base pair at an approximate frequency of one in 200–500 base pairs as a normal variation. When the single base change occurs in a restriction site (where specific restriction endonucleases cut the consecutive sequence specific for each enzyme), the restriction fragments resulting from digestion by the enzyme include fragments of different length at the region concerned (length polymorphism). This permits the identification of individual DNA fragments derived from the two homologous chromosomes.

RFLP ANALYSIS OF TUMOUR AND MATCHED NORMAL DNA

Paired tumour and adjacent normal tissues or, alternatively, peripheral blood leukocytes, are obtained. High-molecular-weight genomic DNA is extracted from snap-frozen tissues. Genomic DNA is cut by specific endonucleases into a huge number of small DNA pieces and then separated according to the size of restriction fragments on an agarose gel. The fractionated DNA is subsequently transferred onto nylon membranes and the individual DNA fragments can be identified by hybridizing with well-mapped and radiolabelled exogenous human DNA sequences (DNA probes). Thus restriction fragments (known as alleles) complementary to the DNA probe are demonstrated as autoradiographic signals.

It gives two allele signals of different size on autoradiogram if length polymorphism exists between two restriction fragments, both of which were complementary to the DNA probe examined (heterozygous locus). In contrast, a homozygous locus shows an unique allele as a single signal but with double intensity (Fig. 20.1). When one of the two homologous chromosomal loci are shown to be lost (loss of heterozygosity) in tumour DNA on RFLP analysis, it suggests, as shown in retinoblastomas, that the counterpart locus harbours an inactivated TSG(s). By determining the chromosomal loci showing loss of heterozygosity in tumour DNA, chromosomal regions possibly possessing an inactivated form of TSG are identified.

ALLELOTYPE

By using a panel of DNA probes mapped on each arm of non-acrocentric chromosomes, a picture of the tumour genome can be obtained that demonstrates at the molecular level whether or not loss of genetic information has occurred which could be associated with inactivation of a TSG(s). Such an analysis characterizes the tumour genome in terms of 'allelotype', in contrast to classical 'karyotype' (Vogelstein et al 1989). It also provides the first step in the identification of possible TSGs.

ALLELOTYPE OF UROTHELIAL AND PROSTATIC CANCERS

In the present study, clinical materials obtained at surgical intervention of 11 transitional cell carcinomas of the renal pelvic urothelium (all primary tumours) and 18 adenocarcinomas of the prostate (10 primary tumours,

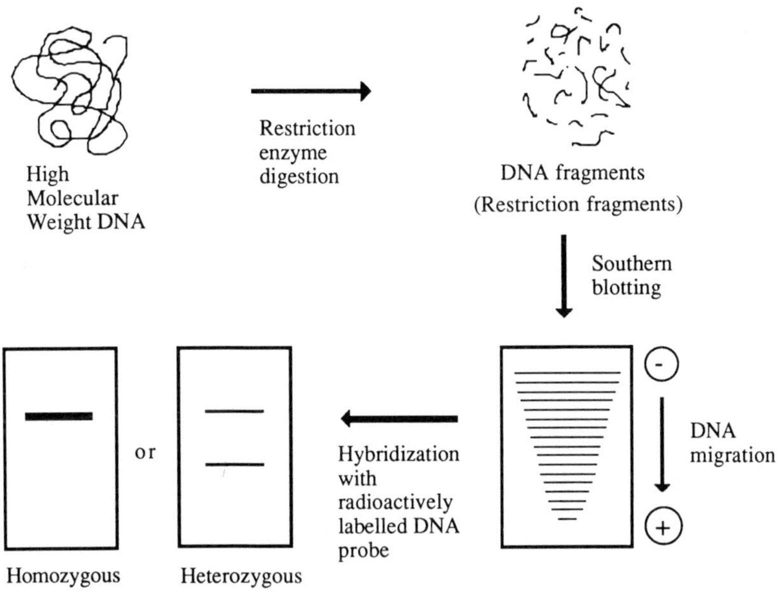

Fig. 20.1 Methodological strategies in RFLP analysis.

four lymph node metastases, and four brain metastases) were surveyed. A total of 54 DNA probes were used in RFLP analysis to cover all areas of the genome; each probe is mapped to a particular part of a chromosome with a minimum of one DNA probe in each arm except for the short arms of chromosomes 13, 14, 15, 21 and 22 (acrocentric chromosomes). Representative Southern autoradiograms are shown in Figs 20.2 and 20.3.

UROTHELIAL CANCER

In urothelial cancers, all of 11 primary tumours studied showed loss of heterozygosity on at least one chromosomal region including either chromosomes 17, 11, or 9, although loss of heterozygosity was widely distributed in several chromosomal regions (Kunimi 1991). Loss of heterozygosity was detected on 17p (73% of informative cases), 11p (64%) and 9p (40%). Loss of genetic information on these chromosomal arms is considered to be of key importance in the oncogenesis of urothelial cancers.

Among seven cases of grade II tumours, the average number of chromosomal arms with allelic losses was 2.57 (range 1–5), whereas four cases of grade III tumours gave an average value of 5.00 (range 2–9) (Table 20.1).

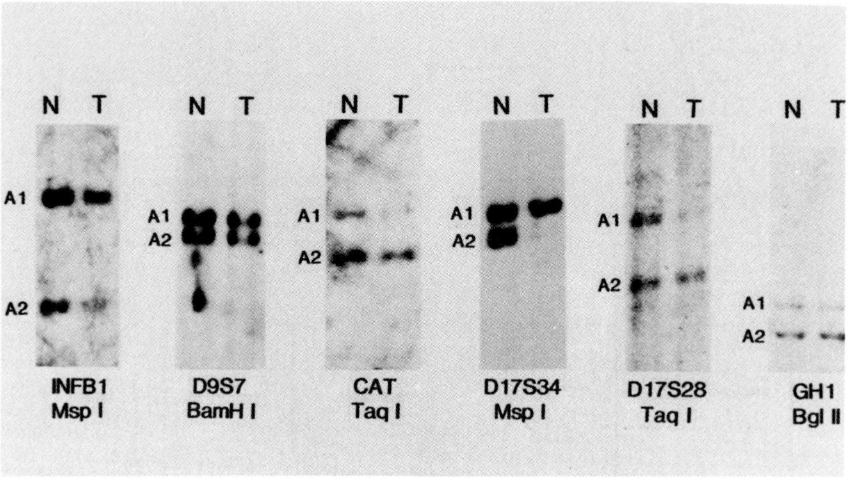

Fig. 20.2 Loss and retention of heterozygosity in an individual urothelial cancer. The restriction enzymes and DNA probes used are indicated at the bottom of each autoradiogram. Note loss of the INFB1 (mapped on 9p) allele A2, the CAT (11p) allele A1, the D17S34 (17p) allele A2 and the D17S28 (17p) allele A1. Both A1 and A2 alleles of the D9S7 (9q) and GH1 (17q) loci are heterozygous in normal (N) and tumour (T) DNA.

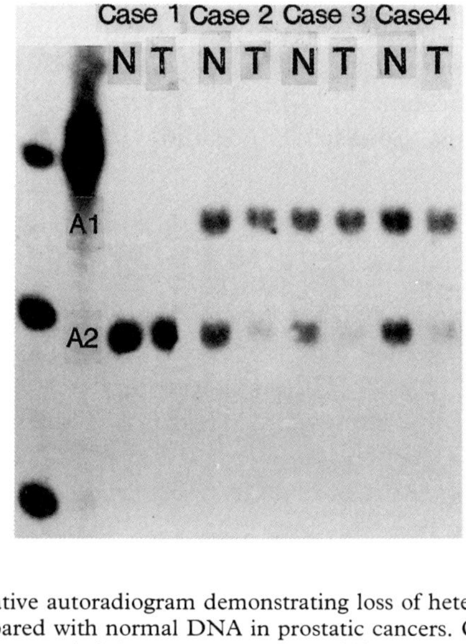

Fig. 20.3 Representative autoradiogram demonstrating loss of heterozygosity on 8p in tumour DNA as compared with normal DNA in prostatic cancers. One of A1 or A2 allele is deleted (loss of heterozygosity) in cases 2, 3 and 4, while case 1 shows homozygosity. The restriction enzyme used is Taq I and the NEFL probe was hybridized. The left two lanes are size marker signals.

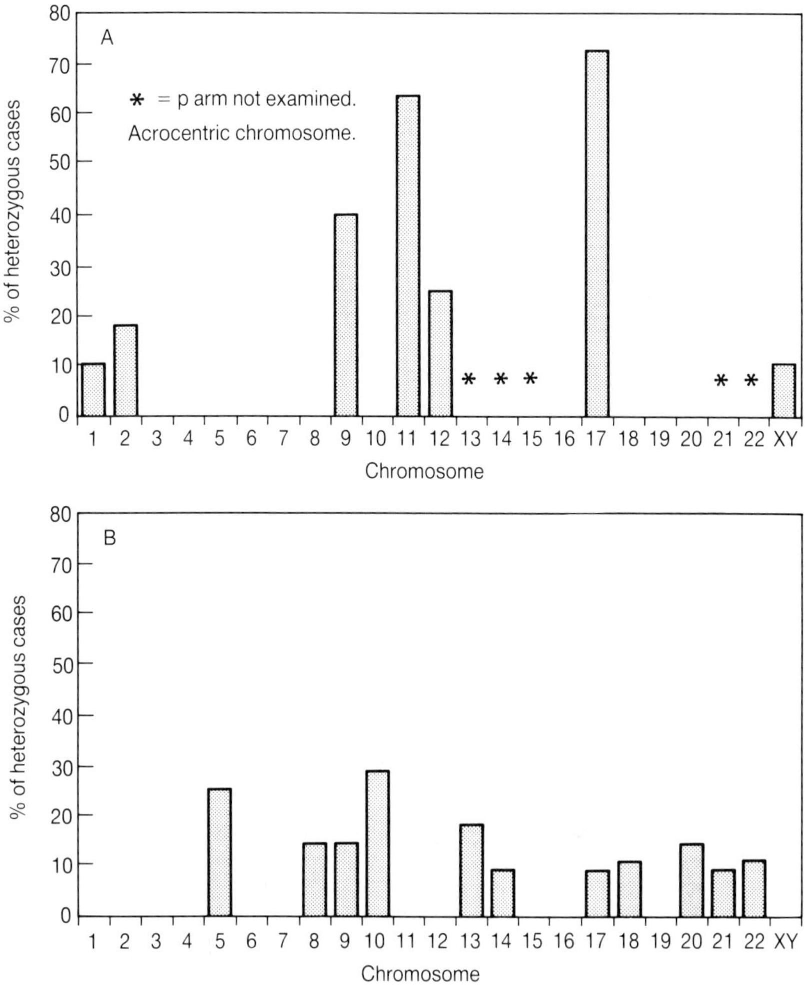

Fig. 20.4 Allelotype of urothelial cancers. **A** p arm. **B** q arm.

Table 20.1 Relationship between the number of chromosomal loci deleted and tumour grade in urothelial cancers

Grade	No. of cases	No. of loci lost Average	Range
II	7	2.57	1–5
III	4	5.00	2–9

PROSTATIC CANCER

In 18 prostatic cancers, 15 of the cases (83%) showed at least one allelic loss on either chromosome 8, 16 or 10 (Kunimi et al 1991). As mentioned

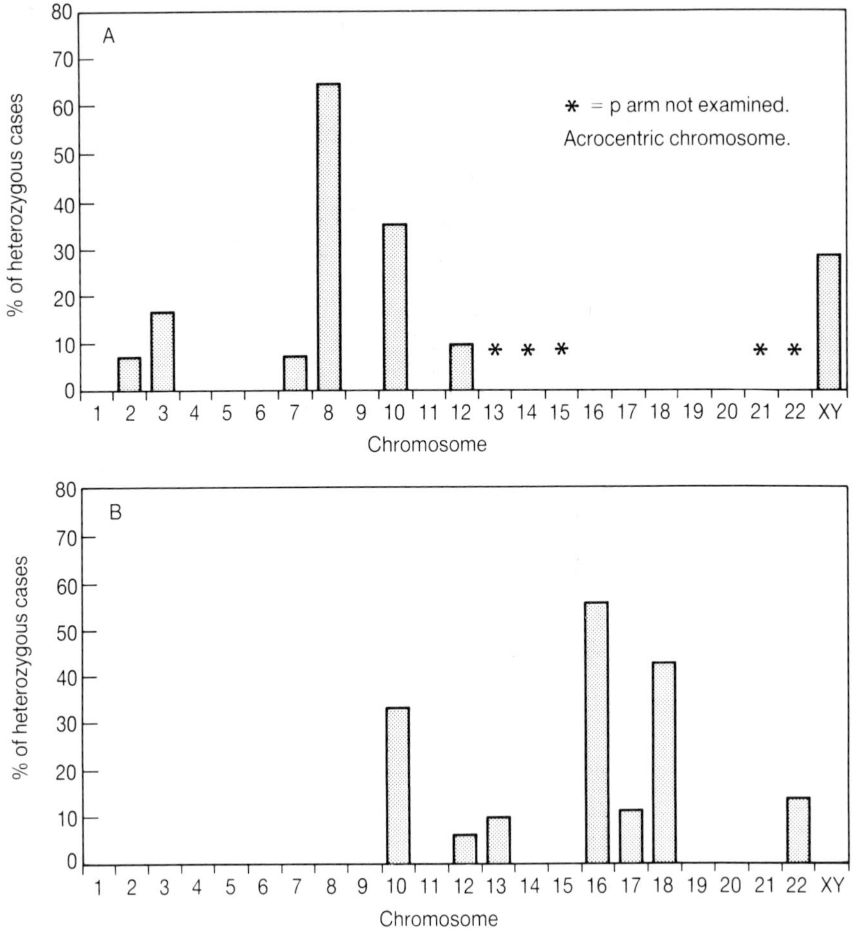

Fig. 20.5 Allelotype of prostatic cancers. **A** p arm. **B** q arm.

above, these chromosomal loci seem likely to harbour inactivated forms of possible TSGs thought to be involved in the oncogenesis of prostatic cancers. Nonrandom allelic losses were detected on the short arm (p) of chromosome 8 (65% of informative cases), the long arm (q) of chromosome 16 (56%), chromosome 10pq (55%) and 18q (43%) (Fig. 20.5).

In 10 cases of well-differentiated adenocarcinomas, the average number of allelic losses was 1.00 (range 0–4); nine of these cases showed 0.33 allelic losses, with one brain metastasis case with a value of four. In contrast the average value in eight poorly differentiated cases was 2.63 (range 0–6). Ten primary tumours, four lymph node metastases, and four brain metastases gave the value of 0.33 (range 0–1), 2.00 (range 2), and 4.00 (range 1–6),

Table 20.2 Relationship between number of chromosomal loci deleted and tumour grade and clinical stage

	No. of cases	No. of loci lost Average	Range
Grade			
Highly differentiated	10	1.00	0–4
	(1 case brain metastases)	4	4
	(9 cases)	0.33	0–1
Poorly differentiated	8	2.63	0–6
Stage			
Primary	10	0.70	0–4
	(1 case, poorly differentiated)	4	4
	(9 cases)	0.33	0–1
Lymph node metastases	4	2.00	2
Brain metastases	4	4.00	1–6

respectively (Table 20.2). In both prostatic and urothelial cancers, the higher grade and stage tumours tended to show more allelic losses.

GENETIC BACKGROUND OF UROGENITAL CANCERS

LOSS OF HETEROZYGOSITY

The present RFLP data indicate that losses of gene products or their functions have occurred in both forms of urological tumour and are thus probably involved in the oncogenesis, as demonstrated in other diverse human tumour types. Through molecular genetic analysis of, for example, retinoblastomas and colorectal carcinomas, Rb1, p53 and DCC genes have been identified as TSGs from the deleted regions. Possible TSGs can thus be tentatively located on chromosomal regions with allelic losses, where recessive inactivational events have probably occurred to provide the malignant phenotypes. Alternatively, the deleted areas may not represent a second mutation of the residual allele; rather, a reduction in gene dosage may contribute to the oncogenesis.

POSSIBLE TSGs

The growing number of chromosomal loci found by RFLP analysis to be deleted in a variety of human tumours may correspond to a pool of possible TSGs, partly identified. The inactivation of certain TSGs has been widely detected in different types of tumours with varying frequencies, while other TSGs are inactivated in some specific tumour type.

Since 17p loss has been reported to be associated with recessive mutations of the P53 gene (mapped on 17p13), the inactivation of the P53 gene product may also play a role in the oncogenesis of urothelial cancers. By sequencing the residual copy of the gene, we have found that the remaining allele harbours point mutations in the highly conserved exonal regions of the p53 gene (Kunimi et al 1991, submitted for publication).

8p loss in prostatic cancers was karyotypically observed in in vitro LNCaP androgen-unresponsive sublines, although the androgen-responsive sublines showed no 8p loss (Koning et al 1989). The genetic alteration suggests that 8p loss, or alternatively tentative TSG(s) located in the area, may be crucial to androgen-responsive growth.

16q loss has been reported in breast cancers (Larsson et al 1990) as well as in karyotypes of in vitro prostatic cancer cell lines (Lundgren et al 1988). There is, therefore, a possibility that 16q loss could participate in hormonal growth due to the presence in this region of an as yet unidentified TSG(s).

GENETIC COMPLEXITY IN FULLY TRANSFORMED PHENOTYPE

Our data indicate that clinically more aggressive tumours show greater number of chromosomal regions with allelic losses. As clearly demonstrated in colorectal cancer (Vogelstein et al 1988) and glioblastomas (James et al 1988), the development of normal cells into fully malignant cells through the premalignant stages requires stepwise genetic alterations, including the aberrations of oncogenes and TSGs. This phenomenon could supply a new criterion of pathogenesis of cancers in terms of genetic background.

PERSPECTIVES

A more detailed mapping of the minimal consistently deleted regions will narrow down the number of TSG candidates to be investigated. We have reported deletion mapping analysis in prostatic cancer by increasing the number of DNA probes on the chromosomes concerned (Bergerheim et al 1991). This may define the area of interest and facilitate the isolation of the TSG(s).

The discovery of TSGs as well as oncogenes in in-vivo tumours has added a new dimension to our understanding of pathogenesis in cancers. In conjunction with the new molecular genetic techniques, knowledge of the genotype of cancer cells has great diagnostic and therapeutic potential.

ACKNOWLEDGEMENTS

This work was done in a series of cooperative research projects between the Department of Urology, Karolinska Hospital, Sweden and the Department of Urology, Kanazawa University Hospital, Japan.

REFERENCES

Benedict W F, Banerjee A, Mark C et al 1983 Non-random chromosomal changes in direct preparations of primary retinoblastoma. Cancer Genet Cytogenet 10: 311–333
Bergerheim U S R, Kunimi K, Collins V P et al 1991 Deletion mapping of chromosomes 8, 10, and 16 in human prostatic carcinoma. Genes Chromosom Cancer 3: 215–220
Bookstein R, Shew J Y, Chen P L et al 1989 Suppression of tumorigenicity of human prostatic carcinoma cells by replacing a mutated RB gene. Science 247: 712–715
Cavenee W K, Dryja T P, Phillips R A et al 1983 Expression of recessive alleles by chromosomal mechanisms in retinoblastoma. Nature 305: 779–784
Cavenee W K, Hansen M F 1988 Molecular genetics of human familial cancer. Cold Spring Harbor Symposia on Quantitative Biology LI: 829–835
Cossman J 1990 Molecular genetics in cancer diagnosis. Elsevier Science Publishing, New York
Fearon E R, Cho K R, Nigro J M et al 1990 Identification of a chromosome 18q gene that is altered in colorectal cancers. Science 247: 49–56
Friend S H, Bernards R, Rogelj S 1986 A human DNA segment with properties of the gene that predisposes to retinoblastoma and osteosarcoma. Nature 323: 643–646
Friend S H, Horowitz J M, Gerber M R et al 1987 Deletions of a DNA sequence in retinoblastomas and mesenchymal tumors. Proc Nat Acad Sci USA 84: 9059–9063
Green A R 1988 Recessive mechanisms of malignancy. Br J Cancer 58: 115–121
Harris H, Miller O J, Klein G et al 1969 Suppression of malignancy by cell fusion. Nature 223: 363–368
Huang H-J S, Yee J-K, Shew J-Y 1988 Suppression of the neoplastic phenotype by replacement of the RB gene in human cancer cells. Science 242: 1563–1566
James C D, Carlbom E, Dumanski J P 1988 Clonal genomic alterations in glioma malignancy stages. Cancer Res 48: 5546–5551
Knudson A G 1971 Mutation and cancer: statistical study of retinoblastoma. Proc Nat Acad Sci USA 68: 820–823
Knudson A G, Meadows A T, Nichols W W et al 1976 Chromosomal deletion and retinoblastoma. New Engl J Med 295: 1120–1123
Koning J J, Kamst E, Hagenmeijer A 1989 Cytogenetic characterization of several androgen responsive and unresponsive sublines of the human prostatic carcinoma cell line LNCaP. Urol Res 17: 79–86
Kunimi K, Hisazumi H, Collins V P 1991 Point mutations of the TP53 gene in urological cancers. AUA Annual Meeting 86, Abstract 399
Kunimi K, Bergerheim U S R, Larsson I L et al 1991 Allelotyping of human prostatic adenocarcinomas. Genomics 11, in press
Kunimi K, Uchibayashi T, Hisazumi H 1991 Oncogene amplification and inactivation of tumor suppressor genes in urological tumors: the application of restriction fragment length polymorphism analysis. Jpn J Urol 82, in press
Kunimi K, Collins V P 1991 p53 point mutations in urothelial and renal cancers. Submitted for publication
Larsson C, Bystrom C, Skoog L et al 1990 Chromosomal mutations in human breast cancer genes, chromosomes and cancer 2: 191–197
Lundgren R, Kristoffersson U, Heim S et al 1988 Multiple structural chromosome rearrangements including del (7p) and del (10q) in an adenocarcinoma of the prostate. Cancer Genet Cytogenet 35: 103–108
Nigro J M, Baker S J, Preisinger A C et al 1989 Mutations in the p53 gene occur in diverse human tumour types. Nature 342: 705–708
Sager R 1989 Tumor suppressor gene: the puzzle and the promise. Science 246: 1406–1412
Sidransky D, Von Eschenbach A, Tsai Y C et al 1991 Identification of p53 gene mutations in bladder cancer and urine samples. Science 252: 706–709
Vogelstein B, Fearon E R, Hamilton S R et al 1988 Genetic alterations during colorectal tumor development. N Engl J Med 319: 525–532
Vogelstein B, Fearon E R, Kern S E 1989 Allelotype of colorectal carcinoma. Science 244: 207–211

21. The oncogenic human papillomavirus types 16 and 18 are not involved in human prostate carcinogenesis

P. J. Effert R. A. Frye A. Neubauer E. T. Liu P. J. Walther

INTRODUCTION

The association of human papillomavirus (HPV) with human carcinomas (particularly tumours of the genital tract) is well established. There is experimental evidence of the oncogenic potential of HPVs, particularly types 16 and 18. HPV 16 DNA transforms NIH-3T3 cells in the classical transformation assay (Yasumoto et al 1986). Furthermore, integrated HPV 16 or HPV 18 sequences have been detected in tissue from many primary as well as metastatic cervical carcinomas. Also, most cell lines derived from cervical cancer (HeLa, SiHa, CaSki) contain such sequences.

While little is known about the molecular events relevant to prostate carcinogenesis, evidence from several epidemiologic studies appears to support the concept of a sexually transmissible agent being a factor in the development of prostate cancer (Morriseau et al 1970, Wynder et al 1971, Feminella & Lattimer 1973). Recent evidence has demonstrated that HPV can infect the male genital tract; such infections have been localized to the external genitalia and urethra (Levine et al 1984). Seminal fluids from patients with disseminated cutaneous HPV infections were also found to contain HPV DNA. Further evidence of the potential role of HPV types 16 and 18 in the causation of human prostate cancer was provided by recent studies by McNicol and Dodd. Initially, in a limited study, they reported the detection of HPV 16 DNA in a substantial number of benign and all of four malignant prostate tumours (McNicol & Dodd 1990). In an expanded series, 13/27 prostate cancer specimens were found to contain HPV 16 (McNicol & Dodd 1991). If confirmed, these findings could lead to an important new approach in prostate cancer control (particularly in regard to cancer screening). However, *all* prostate cancer specimens analyzed by McNicol and Dodd had been obtained by transurethral resection, and tissue might thus have been contaminated by virally infected urethral cells. We sought to re-address this critical issue by devising a rigorous strategy: a series of 30 paraffin-embedded prostate cancer specimens exclusively obtained by radical prostatectomy was analyzed by modifications of the polymerase chain reaction. PCR-based analysis of paraffin-embedded specimens is a well established technique (Shibata 1988, Claas 1989). While maintaining high sensitivity in the detection of target DNA, it also allows for dissection of microscopically identified cancerous regions. Consequently, urethral mucosa and benign prostatic hyperplasia nearly uniformly found in older males can be excluded from analysis. Furthermore, the use of 'differential PCR' (D-PCR) (Frye et al 1989) for our study, involving co-amplification of both a reference gene and a target HPV-sequence, allows semiquantitative assessment of target gene-copy number. In our experience, the high risk of laboratory contamination from DNA-crossover is also substantially reduced with this technique.

MATERIALS AND METHODS

Tissues

Paraffin-embedded tissue blocks from 30 radical prostatectomy, specimens were selected to include a spectrum of morphological grades. Each block was cut with a fresh, uncontaminated blade, and cancerous regions were identified by a pathologist on the corresponding tissue sections. Areas harbouring greater than 80% malignant cells were demarcated from single 8–10 μM sections, placed directly into the PCR-reaction tubes and deparaffinized (one wash in xylene, two washes in absolute ethanol). Similarly, eight paraffin-embedded cervix carcinoma specimens were randomly chosen and processed in the same manner.

Cell lines

Human cervical carcinoma cell lines SiHa (1–2 copies of HPV 16) and HeLa (10–50 copies of HPV 18), after resuspension in 1% agarose, were subjected to the identical fixation- and paraffin-embedding protocol as was used for the prostate and cervix carcinoma specimens. After deparaffinization, single 8-μm sections of the respective cell lines subsequently served as positive controls in the PCR-reactions.

PCR-amplification

Oligonucleotide primer pairs were chosen to amplify 99- and 88-base-pair sequences within the E6-gene of HPV 16 and 18, respectively. A 150-base-pair fragment of the human gamma-interferon gene was coamplified in each PCR-reaction and served as an internal control. The PCR was performed for 35 cycles under standard conditions in a Perkin-Elmer Cetus thermocycler (94°C denaturation, 50°C annealing, 72°C extension). After PCR, one tenth of the amplified products was visualized by ethidium bromide staining after electrophoresis on 12% polyacrylamide gels.

Southern blot hybridization

Amplification products were electrophoresed on 4% agarose gels and subsequently transferred to 'Hybond-N' nylon filters to which the oligonucleotide probes (representing regions internal to the amplified HPV sequences) were added. After an overnight hybridization at 37°C, filters were washed in succession with 6×SSC at room temperature, TMAC-buffer at room temperature and TMAC-buffer at 58°C. Autoradiography was performed at −70°C for up to 48 hours using an intensifying screen.

RESULTS AND DISCUSSION

After establishing the appropriate PCR-conditions, the HPV type specificity of our primer pairs could be confirmed. The 150-bp gamma interferon reference gene band, present in a single copy in each cell, was coamplified in all the samples, confirming adequate DNA quality.

Compared to other currently available detection systems, PCR-based assays offer the highest sensitivity for the detection of viral infections in tissue samples (Schneider 1989). These assays can be applied to formalin-fixed, archival tissues, thus allowing for rapid accrual of study samples and easy selection of certain populations of cells (e.g. cancer vs. normal cells). The sensitivity of our detection system, determined by progressively diluting SiHa-DNA (1–2 copies of HPV 16) with 'normal' DNA not containing any HPV-sequences, was found to be at the 5% level by ethidium bromide staining (mimicking a hypothetical situation where only 5 of 100 cancer cells in a tissue section harboured 1–2 copies of the HPV-16 sequence). Southern hybridization of this dilution series further increased the sensitivity at least to the 1% level.

Cancerous areas from 30 prostate adenocarcinoma specimens in archival surgical pathological blocks were localized and dissected excluding urethral mucosa. When analyzed by D-PCR, none of the tumours was found to contain detectable sequences of either HPV 16 or HPV 18. These negative results were further confirmed by Southern hybridization of the corresponding samples using HPV-type-specific gene probes. In contrast, both HPV 16 and HPV 18 were detected in 2 out of 8 randomly chosen archival cervical carcinoma specimens using the 'D-PCR' methodology.

These findings are in marked contrast to the PCR data obtained by McNicol and Dodd, where the majority of prostate cancer specimens analyzed were found to contain HPV 16 (McNicol & Dodd 1990, McNicol and Dodd 1991). Different target sequences cannot account for these discordant findings, since the primers used by McNicol and Dodd also targeted the E6 gene of HPV. It appears more likely that the discordance of results may be a problem of tissue sampling. All malignant prostate tissues analyzed by McNicol and Dodd were obtained by transurethral resection and thus were potentially contaminated by HPV-colonized urethral mucosa. In fact, McNicol and Dodd themselves acknowledged that a microdissection approach as used in our study might be critical in order to specifically determine association of the virus with actual prostate cancer tissue (McNicol & Dodd 1991).

The data also highlight another potential drawback of PCR-studies based on *single* target gene amplification – the high risk of contamination. We have found that in D-PCR, the probability of carry-over contamination is significantly reduced since, by coamplification of a target gene with a reference gene, the gene sequence present in relative abundance in the PCR-reaction is preferentially amplified. Furthermore, because of its high sensitivity (it can detect HPV sequences at the 1% level when performed in conjunction with Southern hybridization), D-PCR would appear to be extremely suitable for this application. Although single gene PCR may be somewhat more sensitive, the presence of HPV sequences at less than one copy in 100 cells would be of questionable significance in a clonally derived malignant process. It is therefore concluded that the lack of detection of the critical E6 DNA sequences of HPV 16 and 18 in cancerous cells of radical prostatectomy specimens argues against any significant involvement of these putatively oncogenic HPV types in human prostate carcinogenesis. Larger cancer control epidemiological studies to assess risk of development of prostate cancer in individuals infected by HPV 16 or HPV 18 would appear highly premature and at this time unlikely to be indicated.

REFERENCES

Claas E C, Melchers W J, Van Der Linden H C et al 1989 Human papillomavirus detection in paraffin-embedded cervical carcinomas and metastases of the carcinomas by the polymerase chain reaction. Am J Path 135: 703–709

Feminella J, Lattimer J K 1973 An apparent increase in genital carcinomas among wives of men with prostatic cancer. Pirquet Bulletin of Clinical Medicine 20: 3

Frye R A , Benz C C, Liu E T 1989 Detection of amplified oncogenes by differential polymerase chain reaction. Oncogene 4: 1153

Levine R, Crum C, Herman E et al 1984 Cervical papillomavirus infection and intraepithelial neoplasia: a study of male sexual partners. Obstet Gynecol 64: 16

McNicol P J, Dodd J G 1990 Detection of human papillomavirus DNA in prostate gland tissue by using the polymerase chain reaction amplification assay. J Clin Microbiol 28: 409–412

McNicol P J, Dodd J G 1991 High prevalence of human papillomavirus in prostate tissues. J Urol 145: 850–853

Morriseau P M, Phillips C A, Leadbetter G W 1970 Viral prostatitis. J Urol 103: 767

Schneider A 1989 What are the various methods for HPV detection? Diagn Cytopathol 5: 339–341

Shibata D K, Arnheim N, Martin W J 1988 Detection of human papilloma virus in paraffin-embedded tissue using the polymerase chain reaction. J Exp Med 167: 225–230

Wynder E L, Mabuchi K, Whitmore W F 1971 Epidemiology of cancer of the prostate. Cancer 28: 344

Yasumoto S, Burkhardt A L, Doniger J 1986 Human papillomavirus type 16 DNA-induced malignant transformation of NIH 3T3 cells. J Virol 57: 572–577

Index